Volume 04
Issue 03
November 2009

The Senses & Society

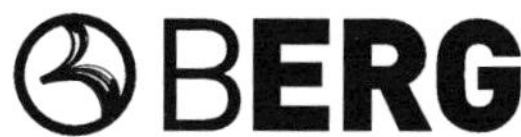

AIMS AND SCOPE

A heightened interest in the role of the senses in culture and society is sweeping the human sciences, supplanting older paradigms and challenging conventional theories of representation.

This pioneering journal provides a crucial forum for the exploration of this vital new area of inquiry. Peer-reviewed and international, it brings together groundbreaking work in the humanities and social sciences and incorporates cutting-edge developments in art, design, and architecture. Every volume contains something for and about each of the senses, both singly and in all sorts of novel configurations.

Sensation is fundamental to our experience of the world. Shaped by culture, gender, and class, the senses mediate between mind and body, idea and object, self and environment. The senses are increasingly extended beyond the body through technology, and catered to by designers and marketers, yet persistently elude all efforts to capture and control them. Artists now experiment with the senses in bold new ways, disrupting conventional canons of aesthetics.

- **How is perception shaped by cultures and technologies?**
- **In what ways are the senses sites for the production and practice of ideologies of gender, class, and race?**
- **How many senses are there to "aesthetics"?**
- **What are the social implications of the increasing commercialization of sensation?**
- **How might a focus on the cultural life of the senses yield new insights into processes of cognition and emotion?**

The Senses & Society aims to:

- Explore the intersection between culture and the senses
- Promote research on the politics of perception and the aesthetics of everyday life
- Address architectural, marketing, and design initiatives in relation to the senses
- Publish reviews of books and multi-sensory exhibitions throughout the world
- Publish special issues concentrating on particular themes relating to the senses

To submit an article, please write to David Howes at:

The Senses and Society
Department of Sociology and Anthropology
Concordia University
1455 de Maisonneuve Ouest
Montreal, Quebec
Canada H3G 1M8

email:
senses@alcor.concordia.ca

Books for review should be sent to Boris Wiseman at:

Boris Wiseman
Copenhagen University,
Department of English, German and Romance Studies
Njalsgade 128
DK-2300
Copenhagen
Denmark

email:
b.wiseman@hum.ku.dk

Suggestions regarding Sensory Design reviews should be addressed to Medina Lasansky

email:
DML34@Cornell.edu

Suggestions regarding Multisensory Exhibition and Conference reviews should be addressed to Jim Drobnick

email:
jdrobnick@faculty.ocad.ca

©2009 Berg. All rights reserved. No part of this publication may be reproduced or utilized in any form or by any means, electronic or mechanical, including photocopying and recording, or by any information storage or retrieval system, without permission in writing from the publisher.

ISSN (print): 1745-8927
ISSN (online): 1745-8935

The Senses and Society is indexed by: Abstracts in Anthropology; AOI Anthropological Index Online; ARTbibliographies Modern; Art Index; British Humanities Index; DAAI Design and Applied Arts Index; IBSS International Bibliography of the Social Sciences; IBR (International Bibliography of Book Reviews of Scholarly Literature in the Humanities and Social Sciences); IBZ (International Bibliography of Periodical Literature in the Humanities and Social Sciences); MLA International Bibliography; Scopus; Sociological Abstracts

Berg Publishers is a member of CrossRef

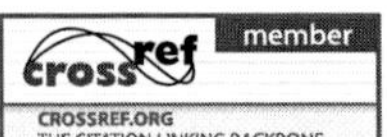

SUBSCRIPTION INFORMATION

Three issues per volume.

One volume per annum.

2009: Volume 4

ONLINE
www.bergpublishers.com

BY MAIL
Berg Publishers
C/o Customer Services
Turpin Distribution
Pegasus Drive
Stratton Business Park
Biggleswade
Bedfordshire SG18 8TQ
UK

BY FAX
+44 (0)1767 601640

BY TELEPHONE
+44 (0)1767 604951

BY EMAIL
custserv@turpin-distribution.com

INQUIRIES

Julia Hall, Managing Editor
email: jhall@bergpublishers.com

Production: Ken Bruce, email: kbruce@bergpublishers.com

Advertising and subscriptions: Corina Kapinos, email: ckapinos@bergpublishers.com

SUBSCRIPTION RATES

Print

Institutional: (1 year) $358/£184; (2 year) $573/£294

Individual: (1 year) $70/£40*; (2 year) $112/£64*

Online only

Institutional and individual: (1 year) $305, £156; (2 year) $487, £250

*This price is available only to personal subscribers and must be prepaid by personal cheque or credit card

Free online subscription for institutional print subscribers

Full color images available online

Access your electronic subscription through www.ingentaconnect.com

REPRINTS FOR MAILING

Copies of individual articles may be obtained from the publishers at the appropriate fees.
Write to

Berg Publishers
1st Floor, Angel Court
81 St Clements Street
Oxford OX4 1AW
UK

The Senses and Society is hosted by the Faculty of Arts and Sciences, Concordia University. The Editors wish to express their thanks for Concordia's support.

Typeset by JS Typesetting Ltd, Porthcawl, Mid Glamorgan
Printed in the UK

The Senses & Society

**Volume 04
Issue 03
November 2009**

Contents

Articles

Design Review

Book Reviews

Exhibition Reviews

Senses & Society   **VOLUME 4, ISSUE 3**   **REPRINTS AVAILABLE**   **PHOTOCOPYING**   **© BERG 2009**
                         PP 273–282   **DIRECTLY FROM THE**   **PERMITTED BY**   **PRINTED IN THE UK**
                                                      PUBLISHERS   **LICENSE ONLY**

The Voices of Things

Alphonso Lingis

Alphonso Lingis is Professor of Philosophy at the Pennsylvania State University. His books include *Excesses: Eros and Culture, The Community of Those Who Have Nothing in Common, Abuses, The Imperative, Dangerous Emotions, Trust, Body Modifications: Evolutions and Atavisms in Culture*, and *The First Person Singular*.
allingis@hotmail.com

ABSTRACT   We find ourselves summoned forth by the earth, the light, water, and fire; we find ourselves directed by the things about us. Things lure us, provoke us, direct us, charm, or hex us. Animism and fetishism designate two different ways we have understood these experiences. Although a specific form of animism has come to dominate in our art and epistemology, fetishist ontology remains and returns.

KEYWORDS: animism, fetishism, animist art, Marx, Freud

We find ourselves summoned forth by the earth, the light, water, and fire; we find ourselves directed by the things about us. Animism and fetishism designate two different ways we have understood these experiences. Animism – from *animus*, wind, spirit, voice – recognizes a spirit in material things. This spirit is separate from them. The Book of Genesis opens with the Spirit speaking in the void and ordering the waters above and the waters below; seas and dry land; flying and swimming, creeping and crawling things. Yahweh speaks to Moses from the burning bush. In Greece the oracle speaks

Senses & Society   DOI 10.2752/174589209X12464528171815

in the vapors rising from the cleft rock at Delphi. Since the spirit, or spirits, can speak in things anywhere, animism sees our whole environment, living and nonliving, to be a realm of meaning.

The form given to the voice can convey information about things near and far. A voice can also address, call upon, and order us. Our linguistics recognizes the vocative and imperative force of speech acts; our grammar and rhetoric classify their forms and uses. But our sciences, even our psychology, do not account for the fact that a voice uttered at a distance can penetrate to the core of our identity and appeal to us and put demands on us. A child may be ordered by the voice of a parent when he or she is no longer there; an adult may hear that voice when the parent is no longer alive, may hear too the parents of that parent. Indeed, is there any society where the voices of ancestors are utterly silenced? Animism recognizes that voices addressing us and ordering us may be the voices of other species, and voices of the absent and the dead. They can be heard in things.

Fetishism recognizes a silent voice of material things themselves (Pels 1998: 91). Things lure us, provoke us, direct us, charm, or hex us. The voice that is heard is only in this singular material thing, which we come upon by chance. Fetishism recognizes a realm of good and bad luck.

We find ourselves in a partly or largely man-made environment whose structures, tasks, and paths were planned, and we design our actions and follow maps and signs. Yet even there, we encounter nourishing, energizing, and enchanting things and sinister and baleful things by chance. Strokes of good or bad luck, they lead us into byways and freeways from which we may not return to our planned objectives. We plan our day, program our ambitions, diagram our life, but, looking back, we may recognize that the essential turns our life took were determined by chance encounters – a captivating teacher, an opportunity that opened and that brought us to a work we love, someone met by chance who became our lover and life partner, a debilitating accident, a disease. That we were born with our sound or sickly body, with our particular sensibility, that we were born at all, were strokes of luck.

Images of the Fetishist World

In the cave paintings of Chauvet, dated 32,000 BCE, Cosquer, 27,000 BCE, Altamira, 18,500 BCE, and Lascaux, 15,000 BCE, the art has already reached mastery in the expressive use of the supporting rock, the shadings of pigments, the composition of forms, the use of split perspective to put the figures in movement. Pablo Picasso, in viewing these techniques at Lascaux, said, "We have learned nothing in twelve thousand years." Aurochs, bison, tigers, antelopes, horses are portrayed in movement and depicted with astonishing anatomical skill. Yet typically there are no images of humans. In Lascaux there is a stick figure of a man with the head of a bird. In

Chauvet there are none; in Cosquer there is one stick figure of a dead man.

Humans did leave the mark of their hands. In these caves and caves in Patagonia, in the Sahara and the Kalahari, in Indonesia, and in Australia, peoples with no cultural links to each other covered rock walls with stencils of their hands, made by holding their hands to the cave wall and blowing dry or liquid pigment across them. Handprints made by simply dipping one's hand in colored clay and pressing it against the cave wall are rare. Archaeologists are baffled both by the universality of the hand silhouettes found in caves continents apart, and by their possible significance. Should we see in them the impulse to mark inert substance with the mark of human presence and will? But the stencils outline the absence of a hand. The hands vanished, leaving only the rock, or perhaps they vanished into the rock.

There are peoples who never marked and designed the landscape in which they lived. The Maasai of Africa refuse to wound the earth; they do not chop into the ground to plant gardens or fields but instead live off the milk of their cattle and what wild plants they can gather, drawing the blood of bulls – in small quantities so as not to weaken them – to supplement their diet. They do not cut into the earth to make bricks but instead shape their dwellings of dung from their cattle.

The aboriginal Australians find that the contours and hollows of the continent have a melodic form, and capture it in their songs. Having learned the melodies from their parents, they find their way from one end of the continent to the other by following its songlines. They do not mark the land, but find the landscape already marked with traces of events of the Dreamtime. The monolith Uluru, a ruby-red rock 3.6 kilometers long and 348 meters high, is found planted in flat desert that extends for hundreds of kilometers on all sides, as the very heart of the continent. In immemorial silence and repose the rock sleeps – and dreams. It dreams of pythons and scorpions, blue-tongued lizards and wallabies. The Australians have over generations elaborated a dream analysis of its forms, its furrows, and its hollows. There are paintings in many of these sites, some made on the ground and obliterated by dances performed on them, some in caves that are 42,000 years old. The paintings bring out, and care for, the dreams of the sites themselves.

In India the core of the world was seen in concentrated and pure form in the Shiva linga. It is an oval black stone, with three white lines near the top, set in the yoni, a "womb" not into which the "phallus" plunges but out of which it rises. It is associated with Shiva, who dances in a ring of fire the unending dance of creation and destruction. The most sacred Shiva lingas, few in number and celebrated throughout India, are those made in the heavenly Ganga, that luminous cosmic torrent (which Europeans call the Milky way) that Hindus see descending to Earth at Pashupatinath in the Himalayas, where the earthly Ganga, the river Ganges, begins and then travels across the subcontinent to plunge into the ocean and reemerge in the most remote heavens. The most sacred celestial Shiva lingas are found at Pashupatinath. (These celestial Shiva lingas Europeans call meteorites.) The second most sacred Shiva lingas are terrestrial, formed by the river Ganges; they too are few in number. In a cave at Amarnath in Kashmir is found a Shiva linga of ice that reaches its fullest each year in July, and summons tens of thousands of Hindus from all over the subcontinent who come to contemplate it on the night of the full moon. Finally there are the millions of Shiva lingas carved by human hand. On the small island of Gharapuri (Elephanta) off Mumbai there is a cave whose walls have been abundantly carved. On the day of the equinox, the setting sun sends a beam of light that glows on the Shiva linga in the core of the cave. The cosmic and the terrestrial Shiva lingas are primary: in the Hindu conception they could not be images of human genitals "projected" onto them; instead human genitals are tertiary images of them. Rather than marking the human presence in the river plains, the caves, the mountains, and the sky, the Shiva linga marks the human anatomy with the Ganga, the cosmic river.

The Buddhist stupa Borobudur in Java, the greatest monument erected in the southern hemisphere, encloses a small mountain. It is located in the jungle, and you have to take several local buses from Yogyakarta to get there. The time it takes to visit it makes clear what it is doing, and what it is doing to you. As with every stupa, you circumnavigate it clockwise, but here the path rises higher each time spiraling in ten levels as you pass the walls covered with hundreds of bas-reliefs depicting all the activities of humans. As you rise higher and higher up the stupa, the activities depicted become less agitated and more harmonious. You reach the top; there are no more bas-reliefs and you find yourself encircled by seventy-two bell-shaped stupas, whose walls are perforated to show figures of the Buddha inside, but the stupa that is on top at the center is empty, showing nothing, or everything, inside. You look down upon the luxuriant jungle below extending on all sides as far as your eyes can see. To the south the jungle ascends a wall of volcanoes, simmering fumes and shooting out blazing cinders. You find that the concentric circles of the path you have ascended have progressively centered your attention; you find your soul composed, its wayward impulses and desires fade away. The hundreds of images of human activities have brought you back to yourself. But at the summit, there are only the seventy-two figures of the Buddha, there is no longer any individuality seeking to assert itself, neither male nor female, pure postures of cosmic compassion, directing your gaze to the teeming jungle, the fiery volcanoes, and the benevolent sky.

Such works belong to a fetishist world, where it is the voices of things and of the earth, air, water, and fire that summon us and lead us.

The Evolution of Animism

In the Christian West the most revered images were canvases that had been animated by a spirit separated from humans and from the world: Jesus printed his image on the veil of Veronica and on the shroud of Turin. Saint Luke was revered as the artist apostle for having endowed the Church with a painting of Mary, the mother of Jesus. But he was no painter: it was Mary herself who miraculously printed her image on his canvas. Later, in Guadalupe in the New World she printed her image on the mantle of an Aztec peasant named Quauhtlatohua.

When we view the Parthenon in Athens, we are struck by the opposition between the great raw dark rock whose immensurable, incalculable forms were thrust up in some ancient collision of continental plates and the gleaming white construction erected boldly on top of it, a temple determined by the abstract ideas of geometry and housing Athena, Athens represented in a giant human figure. In and around the Parthenon, the primeval forces feared and revered in Greek antiquity, Thunder, Lightning, Fire, Wind, Oceanic Tempest, were contained within human shapes. There, Friedrich Nietzsche said, the Athenians contemplated ideal images of themselves, in which all their passions – for power, for law, for domestic harmony, and loyalty, rage, jealousy, vengefulness, and lust – are affirmed and glorified.

The Renaissance rediscovered the Parthenon and its statues. For the next five hundred years sculptors were at work erecting, in public places all over Europe and then in the European colonies in the Americas, the Indian subcontinent, and Africa, statues of conquerors and rulers depicted in action, their limbs held in significant gestures. The statues are narrative, depicting the ideals Western states and religions have conceived in successive battles and in the foundations of cities, nations, and colonies. They put in inert matter the intentions and achievements of vision, will, resoluteness, and courage. Stone and bronze immobilize these heroic postures, to demonstrate victory over rebellion, disorder, and time.

During the Renaissance Giorgio Vasari recorded how painters introduced perspective, chiaroscuro, and the painted effects of light, and observed too that artists were seen to enhance or modify the religious and cultural ideals depicted and also to introduce ideas of their own. They came to be seen as creators, for the sublime meanings they put in their works were understood to be projections of their creative sensibility and imagination.

In the fifteenth century technological advances used in navigation greatly expanded the conversion of nature into resources and products. European imperialism launched a political and ideological struggle with other cultures. The denunciation of heretical and heathen cultures and of their deities as empty idols attributed the voices heard in them to as the projections of false priests and superstitious peoples.[1] The pidgin word *fetissos*, with which the

Dutch and Portuguese merchants dubbed objects that West Africans kept out of commerce – and that the merchants found valueless and repugnant anyhow – assimilated such objects with *feitiços*, the appurtenances associated with witchcraft in Europe. In the eighteenth century the term "fetish" was taken up by the Enlightenment theory of primitive religion to designate inanimate objects to which "primitives" attribute demonic powers; in the nineteenth century it was taken up by Marx to designate commodities whose exchange value greatly exceeds their use value; and in the twentieth century taken up by Freud to designate objects taken by neurotics as phallic substitutes. This succession of anthropological, sociological, and psychological theories declare that these things are really nothing but what physics and chemistry records of them and that human minds "project" intentions and powers into them. The spirit that speaks in things is not the spirit of ancestors, deities, or alien beings, but our own spirit.[2] These theories are animist explanations of fetishism.

The philosopher Georg Wilhelm Friedrich Hegel, in his *Phenomenology of Spirit*, depicts a great historical movement in which the spirit gradually separates itself from the realm of material things, opposes itself to them, and then takes them over and progressively reshapes the material environment with its desires. The mind finds that it can actively predict how things will react and, guided by its understanding of them, can manipulate them and reshape all things according to its will. The material realm comes to no longer appear indifferent to the spirit, opaque and impenetrable; now the mind recognizes intelligible structures and relations everywhere in things. At a final stage, the mind recognizes that the intelligible structures and relations that we recognize in things are structures and relations that the mind itself has projected into them. The things do not resist these projections, but acquiesce to them. At this stage the spirit recognizes not only that it is separate from the material realm but also that the material realm is not something separate from it but is utterly subject to it; the spirit recognizes its absolute sovereignty.

In 1964 Andy Warhol exhibited "Brillo Box," and launched postmodern art. Artists no longer seek to produce sublime objects, separated from all utility, which would exhibit an ideal meaning. They celebrate coke bottles, soup cans, and blue jeans, which had been taken to have simply utilitarian significance by the advocates of the fine arts. Consumers put meaning in them by defining their identity, status, and happiness with the individual collections they amass and display in their apartments, and with which they network with other collectors of blue jeans, vintage country-western CDs, and baseball cards.

If animism is pushed to the limit, the actual material substance that is animated, that relays the voice of a spirit, can be arbitrary. Yahweh can speak in a burning bush; the spirit of the contemporary world can speak in a coke bottle or a Brillo box. Words have materiality; they have timbre and pitch, attack, accent, and duration. Written words have shape, thickness, size, and color. Postmodern artist Jenny Holzer presents, in commercial lettering or in illuminated neon, not inscribed on things, the political and commercial slogans and catchphrases, cues, watchwords, and passwords by themselves, showing us the messages, the orders, that are incessantly projected about us. The materiality of the words recedes before the agitated and urgent messages being projected upon us by ingenious and calculating human engineering experts and their ironic or provocative variations by Jenny Holzer.

What the artist does, by enshrining these banal and mass-produced things, as also the commercial logos and icons, in art galleries, at this particular time in the evolution of culture, is, philosopher Arthur Danto explains, to show that these consumer products focus and draw our desires for identity, recognition, power, and happiness. The voices of these things are our voices: they are what we have fixed as refreshing, exciting, glamorous, beautiful; they relay the identity and worth we are fashioning for ourselves. Postmodern art represents the moment when artists have become lucidly conscious of themselves and of their activity. It is the moment when – and here Danto invokes Hegel – the spirit becomes self-conscious of its work of interiorizing the exterior (Danto 1992: 9; 1997: 30–3, 66). The moment, we will say, when a universal human animism becomes explicitly conscious of itself.

The specific kind of animism now dominant in our culture – that finds everywhere only the voices we ourselves project into things – would be rooted in a primary urge in humans to mark their presence in things. How frail and ephemeral is our presence in deserts and jungles, in the oceans and under the stormy skies! Would not art first arise in the use of inert material substance – clay, stone, bronze – to maintain enduring the fleeting gestures of life?

The Return of Fetishism

Among the fetishes of Africans and Polynesians found objects – bones, fossils, crystals, burls – are sheathed in often intricately beaded and embroidered pouches or cases. Objects made may also be recognized as fetishes if they are unique or made on the occasion of some chance auspicious event. In 1907 Picasso came upon African fetishes in the ethnographic collections of the Palais de Trocadéro and was captivated by the uncanny power of their forms and designs. Soon he, Braque, Matisse, Derain, Modigliani, and Bréton were acquiring personal collections of them.

If fetishes could be experienced as art, could not artworks be experienced as fetishes? A working artist is not one who has an encyclopedic appreciation of artworks but one who has a passionate devotion to materials and forms that speak singularly to him or her. An artwork emerging in his hands captivates the artist and guides his hand; it goes beyond or goes outside whatever meaning the artist had conceived for it. It beckons him toward unknown paths. Are not artworks so many scattered sites outside the domain of work and reason, in the realm of chance? Are they not so many talismans and omens of good and bad luck? Is there not a factor of luck that makes someone who diligently studies art talented or not? Is there not a factor of luck that determines whether any carving or painting works or does not?

There are in the "art world" individuals who have deliberately cultivated appreciation of artworks of many epochs and styles; they make a living as professional critics and expert advisers to curators and collectors. But for most of us spending an hour or two in the Louvre strangely neutralizes the force of the artworks, producing fatigue. It does seem that the sanctuary, or the home, that has one artwork or a few, with which we live, which unceasingly shapes our sense of the important and the trivial and to which we return, is the normal case. Even experts with an encyclopedic familiarity with artworks often end up writing of one painting or one church that has haunted and directed their lives (Kimmelman 2005).

The form of animism that Arthur Danto identifies as characteristic of our culture finds only our voices in things. But do not our ancestors, do not the dead, do not other living species continually speak to us, summoning us and leading us? A great deal of our art, from our performances of Greek tragic plays to plays and films of the voices of the victims of recent genocides, make us hear the voices of the dead. A major portion of what we have come to call art were rituals and ceremonies celebrating the turning of the seasons and the rebirth of nature after winter or after the dry season and celebrating our relations with other species – the crane dances of Japan and Africa, the totems marking relationship with patron animals. Today we have become aware once again that we share this planet with innumerable other living things, whose voices summon our attention and must also direct our lives. There are today works that do not simply speak to us of our concepts, imagination, values, and pleasures. There is Robert Smithson's *Spiral Jetty*, Donald Judd's *100 Milled Aluminum Boxes*, Michael Heiser's *City*; works made of light, the *Sun Tunnels* of Nancy Holt, Walter de Maria's *Lightning Field*; and works made of air and wind, musique concrète, the random sound assemblages of John Cage.

Are we not today at a turning point in our consciousness and our lives regarding our relationship with the material universe? Molecular chemistry and astronomy have vastly extended the small environment of tools and constructions where we had refashioned a patch of the universe so that it is embedded with our concepts and values. While a postmodern culture and art celebrates, according to Danto, in all things the human desires, conceptions, and pleasures that we project into them, molecular chemistry reveals the things that are in us – analyzing our agitated and contented bodies into chemical compounds suspended in salt water. Could it be that outside inert matter summons and directs our material bodies in ways that biochemists have not yet been able to trace?

We exist on a chunk of rock and minerals whirling about in empty space where we see scattered in the dark voids a few other rock planets and stars, concentrations of fiery gases. We have hardly begun work into our conception of ourselves, our values, and our pleasures, the revelation by astronomy that the sun is burning itself out as fast as it can, and that in another billion years all animal and plant life on Earth, now already 4.5 billion years old, will be incinerated before the exploding end of the sun. We shall have to find a new conception of material reality and recognize the destination and destiny to which it summons us.

Notes

1. But the Europeans, while denouncing idolatry, maintained the animist conviction that spirits speak in victories, miracles, earthquakes – the true spirits of Christ and Saint George, Saint Michael, and Santiago.

2.

   The myths tell us nothing instructive about the order of the world, the nature of reality or the origin and destiny of mankind... They teach us a great deal about the societies from which they originate, they help to lay bare their inner workings and clarify the *raison d'être* of beliefs, customs and institutions...; most importantly, they make it possible to discover certain operational modes of the human mind (Levi-Strauss 1981: 639).

References

Danto, Arthur C. 1992. *Beyond the Brillo Box*. Berkeley: University of California Press.

Danto, Arthur C. 1997. *After the End of Art*. Princeton: Princeton University Press.

Kimmelman, Michael. 2005. *The Accidental Masterpiece*. New York: Penguin.

Lévi-Strauss, Claude. 1981. *The Naked Man*. Trans. John and Doreen Weightman. Chicago: University of Chicago Press.

Pels, P. 1998. "The Spirit of Matter: On Fetish, Rarity, Fact, and Fancy." In Patricia Spyer, ed. *Border Fetishisms: Material Objects in Unstable Spaces*. New York: Routledge.

Senses & Society   VOLUME 4, ISSUE 3   REPRINTS AVAILABLE DIRECTLY FROM THE PUBLISHERS   PHOTOCOPYING PERMITTED BY LICENSE ONLY   © BERG 2009 PRINTED IN THE UK

PP 283–302

The Human Snout: Pigs, Priests, and Peasants in the Parlor

Joseph Nugent

Joseph Nugent received his PhD from UC Berkeley in 2004 and is now an adjunct assistant professor of English at Boston College. He is completing a book manuscript "Between Deference and Devotion: Irish Priests and Irish People." His major upcoming project is a cultural history of smell in nineteenth-century Ireland.
nugentjf@bc.edu

ABSTRACT   Ireland reeked throughout the nineteenth century from the pages of English representation. The reputed stench of its cabins, cesspools, and dungheaps became a shameful index of national backwardness and the essential mark of Irish olfactory identity. In response to the odor of primitiveness that clung to them also, Ireland's rising middle classes set about a program of national decontamination. Led by the emblematic figure of native Victorian propriety, the Catholic priest, this modernizing class carried the mantras of civility and hygiene to the countryside and the rural home, imposing upon a recalcitrant peasantry a new, "enlightened," olfactory register predicated on an intolerance of traditional odors. The groundwork for this

Senses & Society   DOI 10.2752/174589209X12464528171851

transformation was the castigation of Ireland's domestic cottage by English observers and, in particular, the metonymic substitution of the peasantry's pigs for Irish national character – a discursive reordering that, though it encountered resistance from a peasantry devoted to an old Gaelic order of sensory values, was completed and even sanctified by a Catholic Church bent on producing modern, disciplined subjects. The smells of everyday life, as a result, took on new meanings. This paper examines Irish and British literary and historical texts around the turn of the twentieth century to uncover that meaning and expose the role of olfaction in the production of the peculiar Gaelo-Catholic ideology of domesticity that until recent decades governed rural Ireland.

KEYWORDS: smell, Ireland, priest, domestic, civil

"A smell is the most complicated phenomenon in the world," he said, "and it cannot be unraveled by the human snout or understood properly although dogs have a better way with smells than we have."
– "But dogs are very poor riders on bicycles," MacCruiskeen said, presenting the other side of the comparison.

Flann O'Brien

We all know that some nations smell more than others – and certainly more than our own. This is to state merely that national identity contains an olfactory component. The curious case of Ireland will already be known to readers of Jonathan Swift, James Joyce, or Samuel Beckett, whose finely-tuned noses found inspiration in the reek of humanity. Add the lesser-known Flann O'Brien (1911–66) to the list. In his wicked novel *The Poor Mouth* (1941), O'Brien confronts the reader with stench as a cultural, historical, even ideological phenomenon.[1]

The Poor Mouth is set in the fictional village of Corkadorgha in the West of Ireland around the turn of the twentieth century. Its narrator, Bonaparte O'Coonasa, shares a rotting white-washed home with his reputed mother, "a silent, cross, big-breasted woman," and a cantankerous old man of uncertain origin, the Old-Grey-Fellow. The child's mother spends her days endlessly sweeping animal droppings out of the door and boiling housefuls of potatoes for a third inhabitant, Ambrose, the pig that shares their "truly Gaelic" and certainly squalid hovel. When Ambrose was little, Bonaparte recalls, he had a little smell, but now, grown too enormous to exit the front door, he gives off great plumes of what his protector, the Old-Grey-Fellow, calls "pig steam" (O'Brien [1941] 1993: 26). So awful was the stench that "passers-by neither stopped nor even walked when in the vicinity of our house, but raced," says Bonaparte, "past the door" (ibid.: 22). Neighbors, too, were subjected to Ambrose's characteristic scent. Many fled. They "cleared out and went to America," telling people "that Ireland was a fine country but that the air was too strong there" (ibid.: 22).

Smells, O'Brien (and the other great Irish modernists) understood, can make us laugh. Yet, no smell is intrinsically funny; odors have affective power because they are suffused with social meaning, and uncovering that meaning provides new ways to explore how the world is and was. For smells change – rather, smells over time take on new resonances; they elicit varying emotional responses from us, reactions that can, in turn, shape the way we understand and frame our world. Sensory perception, that is, has a role in the construction of ideological frameworks.

The symbolic plane Flann O'Brien chose for his preposterous novel of social satire captures a moment of anxious transition in the modernization of Irish domestic life. The pig in the parlor, badge of all that Ireland was, and the woman's sweeping brush, emblem of what it might be, contend here over the intimate space of the family home – and not just any Irish home, but the whitewashed thatched cottage, later elevated into "a national symbol of an independent, natural, morally upright, and … spiritual way of life" (Kennedy 1993: 173). The kitchen conflict of Corkadorgha enacts two interrelated struggles taking place around the time of the Irish Revival. The greater was an ideological battle between the forces of tradition and modernity; the lesser, a tussle for dominion over domestic space, cast men against women. Both, I want to suggest, were fought to a degree not yet acknowledged over that most elusive and memory-laden sense, the sense of smell.

This paper argues that modern registers of sensory perception were introduced and disseminated by a rising Irish middle class for whom the stench of their peasantry had become a shameful marker of national backwardness. Recoiling from the odor of primitiveness that also clung to them, they demanded that the rural poor cast off practices of animal husbandry and personal hygiene now understood as disgusting. Clergymen were in the van, introducing new notions of personal hygiene and raising the bar of intolerance to traditional odors. The smells of everyday life, as a result, took on new redolence, as the home became a stage – as critics such as Clair Wills (2001) and Joanna Bourke (1993, 1999) have shown – for the enactment of an unequal contest between a pre-bourgeois culture and an emergent ideology of modern domesticity. The effect of this phenomenological transformation was to introduce to a recalcitrant peasantry an olfactory register more akin to European sensibilities and to ease them one step further into modern subjectivity – a reordering that, though it encountered resistance, was completed and even sanctified by the great civilizing force in rural Ireland, the Catholic Church.

A similar alteration in olfactory sensitivity had occurred in France a century before when "something change[d]," Alain Corbin has shown, "in the way smells were perceived and analysed" (1986: 4). While this "olfactory revolution," as the French historian termed it, maps imperfectly onto the peculiarly Catholic Irish experience, clear parallels between the two offer an outline of the olfactory matrix from which this paper emerges. Above all, both experiences, governed by what Norbert Elias called the civilizing process, were articulated as a clash between modernity and tradition. The structural shifts that propelled the French transformation were replicated in Ireland – the spread of an originally urban middle-class sensibility; the codification of a new ideology of domesticity; the dissemination of hygienic discourses from a centralized machinery of state. The cognitive and emotional channels through which this transformation was brought about were also duplicated – odor's deployment as a differentiator of class and an instrument for social discrimination; the heightened awareness of hygiene and the privatization of excrement; the production of disgust at emblematic points of putrefaction, and the consequent arousal of shame. Finally, and very particularly, in both cases there was the perplexing defiance of a peasantry rejecting advances designed, patently, for its betterment.

Smellscape and Character

How strong was the air of Ireland in nineteenth-century literature? Strong enough according to critic James Newcomer, for "whiskey, decay, rot, guttering candles, tobacco damp, horse dung, and dust" (1967: 155) are what lingered in his olfactory imagination after reading the novel with which the century began, Maria Edgeworth's "Big House" novel, *Castle Rackrent* (1800). Nearly a hundred years later it was the decaying cabin that stank. "You want to know," asked George Moore, "what Ireland is like?" "The country exhales," he answered

> the damp, flaccid, evil smell of poverty … it hangs about every cabin; it rises out of the chimney with the smoke of the peat, it broods upon the dung heap and creeps along the deep black bog-holes … the smell of something sick to death of poverty. ([1886] 2004: 19)[2]

In the years between Edgeworth's novel and Moore's diatribe, Ireland reeked from the pages of English representation, for there was, asserts historian Perry Curtis, "scarcely a description of Ireland without its set passage on the dirt, misery, and primitiveness of the Irish cabin or rural dwelling" (1968: 57). To English travelers, that hovel became emblematic of an almost troglodytic people's inability to emerge into the light of modern living. Samuel Carter Hall was horrified by its wretchedness: "A growth of diseased vegetation … mud walls … the pig goes in and out as he pleases," while by the entrance, a "cesspool of stagnant water oozed from the dung-heap" (1883: 482).

"Blurring," in the words of Ina Ferris, "the distinction between earth and habitation," these hovels breached the conceptual walls that Victorians had constructed to keep nature outside of the family home and to protect the precious domesticity within (2002: 35). Affronts to upright English manliness, they were physical expressions of the contorted Irish character, "monuments," sniffed *Punch* in mid-century, "to national idleness," the personification, Dickens thought, of misery (qtd. in Weimer 1993: 360–1). "Happiness," he wrote with sarcasm, "dwelleth in a roofless cabin, with potatoes thrice a week, buttermilk o'Sundays, a pig in the parlour, [and] a fever in the dungheap" (letter to the editor, *Morning Chronicle*, July 25, 1842).

So frequently invoked was the dungheap that the cesspool, that green sink of liquid pig's excrement in which it swam, became the very figure of the wretched island: when Thomas Carlyle returned to Scotland in 1849 he felt, he sighed with relief, as if he were entering "into spring water out of dunghill-puddles" (1882: 441). And emanating from those puddles was what was to become the emblematic smell of Ireland, the whiff of pig manure. In the literature of many, and in the noses of some, that stench dominated what we might term, after geographer J. Douglas Porteus, the "smellscape" of the Irish countryside.

The interior of the Irish cabin held an almost voyeuristic fascination for wandering gentry. George Moore, exploring the recesses of one such, found "a dark place from which exudes a stink; a stink which the inmates describe as a warm smell" ([1867] 2004: 18). There, "a large pig, covered with lice, feeds out of a trough placed in the middle of the floor, and the beast from time to time approaches and sniffs at the child sleeping in a cot by the fireside" (ibid.: 18). It is clear from the nineteenth-century paintings and prints assembled in Claudia Kinmonth's *Irish Rural Interiors in Art* (2006) that the pig Moore observed in the "parlor" was no mere slander but everyday reality.

Remarkably, perhaps, the pig in these illustrations is no intruder. Indeed, the animal is evidently a welcome guest in the domestic space – here sharing a dish of potatoes, there gamboling about the hearth; in one touching cameo an infant snuggles contentedly in the warm embrace of a snoozing, elderly sow.[3] The pig invokes from the family, it seems, none of the disgust that so unsettled their English visitors – or those Irish grandees who, like Moore, now recoiled from the peasantry with a similar distaste. Lady Morgan observed as much in a similar hovel. Sitting down to a plate of sour milk and potatoes she noted a cow "slumber[ing] most amicably with a large pig at no great distance from [me]" (Owenson 1850: 43). Far from distressed with their rank habitation, the family surrounding the playwright were quite content with the "comforts" of their "snug quarters" (ibid.: 43). The Irishman's ease with his pig was at odds, however, with new notions of hygiene already prevailing in England to which, in the latter half of the nineteenth century, the impoverished Irish increasingly fled. But the smell of the pig clung to the Irishman's person – and increasingly came to define his identity.

To the "Little Irelands" of mid-century Liverpool, London, and Glasgow, Friedrich Engels saw them come, bearing their native customs and the noxious odors that accompanied them; like pervasive smells, "these Irishmen … insinuate themselves," he muttered, "everywhere" ([1845] 1942: 91). Pollutants infusing themselves into the body politic, they festered in slums too repellent for all but the intrepid. "Whenever a district is distinguished for especial filth and especial ruinousness," Engels disclosed, the "explorer" may "safely count upon meeting chiefly… Celtic faces" (ibid.: 92). Obtuse, unassimilable, and indifferent to his own stench, "The Milesian continues as he did at home"; he "deposits all garbage and filth before his house door," and "accumulates pools and dirt-heaps" which (Engels now invoking the invisible spirit of *mal aria*) "poison the air" (ibid.: 92). Pools and piles of effluent with their contaminating odors segue comfortably in Engels's mind into images of the pig, and the Irishman, he remarks, "lets the pig sleep in the room with himself" (ibid.: 92). Indeed more, for he "loves his pig," asserts Engels, "as the Arab his horse… He eats and sleeps with it, his children play with it, ride upon it, roll in the dirt with it" (ibid.: 92).

This brand of hostility, some popular journals discovered, could be commercially lucrative. What ensued was a plethora of hostile cartoons in English comic art, comprehensively cataloged by L.P. Curtis in *Apes and Angel* ([1971] 1997). Curtis's genealogy of the protosimian Irishman unearths Paddy's bestial ancestor in James Gillray's United Irishman engravings of the late eighteenth century. In the gaping mouth, upturned nose, exposed nostrils and black marble eyes of these composite creatures we find the visage of the pig. It is as if the Irish body, plainly human in form, must strain to contain a spectral swine struggling to emerge. Fifty years later, the swinish Irish physiognomy continued to issue in the work of George Cruikshank, whose 1845 depictions of Irish brutes "strongly suggest," as Curtis remarks, their "porcine ancestor" ([1971] 1997: 35).

By mid-century, the relationship between Paddy and his pig was firmly and lastingly established. Deeply engrained in the popular English imagination, the animal most closely related to filth and stench continued to metonymically define the Irishman even to the recent past.

Filthy Creatures

There is now a substantial body of scholarship examining the semiotics of the pig, much of it investigating the animal's capacity to evoke in us distaste, even disgust.[4] Peter Stallybrass and Allon White contend that this may be because we in the West, in our long shared history of concord and contention, have invested much in them. Symbolic repositories of the baseness we seek to expunge from our selves but simultaneously desire, they mirror our worst parts. Hapless receptacles of our psychosexual dramas, pigs throughout the ages "seem to have borne the brunt of our rage, fear, affection and desire for the 'low'"; pigs were "creatures of the threshold," "*almost*, but not quite, members of the household" (Stallybrass 1986: 44, 47; emphasis in original).

Indeed not quite, for too much about the pig turns our stomach. For no apparent reason the animal would regularly splash itself in mud or, with evident deliberation and apparent delight urinate in its own dung and wallow in the mix. Avaricious and scandalous, it lurked by latrines in eager anticipation of a feast of human excrement. In contrast to the young of most animals, the piglet was neither lovable nor helpless. Rather, it provided a particularly vicious instantiation for the Victorians of nature, bloody-minded in tooth, if not in claw: armed with razor-sharp eye-teeth it competed from the moment of birth with its siblings, lacerated them, turned on the runt, the most helpless. Even the mother, confounding all natural instincts, was known to consume her own litter.[5]

To be the object of that epithet, "pig," therefore, was to be subjected to a peculiarly demeaning insult. In a world before Porky Pig, Miss Piggy, or Babe, in a time, that is, before commodity capitalism recognized that anthropomorphism could be turned to commercial advantage, that the very identification with the pig that once threatened could now entice, that the pig could be, so to speak, defanged, the affinity with no domestic animal threatened the imperative to civility as did a putative relationship to the pig. In short, the term "pig" functioned as a resonant rhetorical device for marginalization and a catch-all term for those deserving rejection. By association, the pig's doppelgänger, the Irishman, embodied all that was lazy, stupid, unrestrained, dirty, and putrescent.

Distaste for the Irish poor, I have said, crystallized about the emblematic figures of pig and cesspool. These figures, however, are no more than objective correlatives of the underlying emotion that travelers, authors, artists, and even socialists organized about the tropes of health, primitivism, and above all, hygiene. Each of their reports returns us to the sense of smell, for the pig is not offensive to our sight, far less, symbolically, to our Western taste, and the cesspool need not be. Their affective impact – the sense, that is, that reacts to them – is olfaction. Suffused in the multifarious descriptions of the Irish hovel and the piggish Irishman, driving their distaste and emanating through the rhetoric they employ is disgust at the unfragrant pig and its noxious byproducts.

Disgust, Charles Darwin believed, is a universal emotion. His numerous worldwide correspondents saw it expressed and accompanied by a recognizable series of responses – the upper lip retracted, the lower lip protruded, an expiration such as *ach* or *ugh*, the arms tight against the body as we shudder – actions "the same," Darwin observes, as "those we employ when we perceive an offensive odour, and wish to exclude or expel it" ([1872] 1979: 256).[6] Disgust is a universal emotion, but one that seems to be a cultural acquisition. And while it appears to have originated as food rejection, the most potent sensory attribute associated with that "basic" human emotion, experimental psychologists such as Jonathan Haidt and Paul Rozin explain, is odor, specifically the smell of decay and decomposition (Rozin, Haidt, and McCauley 1993: 578–80).[7] They confirm Darwin's observation that this eructive impulse is primarily induced by an assault on our sense of smell. In the facial expression he delineated we see the urge, a primal urge, to recoil and to disgorge from the body the offensive substance we have encountered. Disgust in the nineteenth-century view emblematized by Darwin is a rejection response.[8]

What was to be done? How were the Irish to counteract a representation that exposed, as Stallybrass and White have shown, the dread trace of the abjected other? More immediately, how were they to escape the threat of ejection from the body politic, indeed from the civilized world, implied by the disgust they patently engendered?[9] The Irish middle classes, at least, knew how to respond. Determined not to be contaminated by association with pig and peasant, they appealed directly to the governing classes of England.

Prominent in this rhetorical counterthrust was the Romantic nationalist poet and songwriter Thomas Moore. Writing in the early decades of the nineteenth century, Moore set out to evince from his English drawing-room audiences not disgust but sadness and guilt at an Ireland beautiful but wronged. *In the Morning of Life* is typical of the balladry through which the poet in a tumult of synesthesia petitioned his readers' sensibilities. As the fragrance of Ireland is released by rain falling upon her flowers (Ireland, of course, gendered female), so the sorrowful love that the verse thematizes can, the poem asserts, be "drawn out by tears." Ireland, far from malodorous, Moore asserts in a surfeit of nationalist sentiment, is uniquely fragrant. Indeed, the poem distinguishes his country from those foreign lands where "though splendid the flowers, / Their sighs have no freshness, their odour no worth." In contrast, "'Tis the cloud and the mist of our own Isle of showers / That call the rich spirit of fragrancy forth."

But was Ireland's smellscape, in any but the most wishful sense, fragrant? The answer is, of course, speculative, but may, in fact, be "yes." Outside of its unsewered cities and towns, we should imagine a countryside relatively pleasing to the nose. What filled the nostrils over much of the land were the soft fumes of turf fires – the burning peat to which George Moore refers (above), and with which the Irish cooked and heated until recent decades.[10] The potato crop, whose verdant leaves and delightful purple flower present a gentle fragrance, covered 2.5 million acres (1841 census), 10 percent of the country's land mass. Rural Ireland's problem was not any generalized bad smell; a modern, a quintessentially Victorian, and an eminently English one, it was basically cloacal. Approximately three pounds weight of excrement per day was emitted by each of Ireland's 1.4 million pigs, for whom a third of the land's potato crop was grown (Bourke 1993: 78). The country's predominantly rural population of 8 million people (1841 census) probably produced per capita much the same (pigs and humans consume and eliminate similar volumes).[11] The dungheap by the door was the destination of both these products.

A journey through the smellscape of Ireland, then, we might imagine rather pleasing but interrupted by occasional wafts from the dungheaps befouling the entrance to some peasant hovels. This is hardly sufficient to account for the disgust engendered; that these highly localized instances of odors should so disproportionately offend the English nostril suggests that something else was going on. The disgust they elicited, I suggest, was caused not so much by their presence as their positioning. Disgust, Mary Douglas contends, arises from the breaching of socially demarcated space: things become pollutant by being out of place. Few infractions of spatial propriety were more sure to offend the middle-class Victorian than animal dung in the family home. Victorian ideology had designated that space an olfactory refuge to be carved off with great particularity from the stinks of public life, its kitchen, bosom of domesticity, to be made fragrant by baking, defended by carbolic. The Englishman's disgust at the Irishman's dungheap was caused less by what entered his own nostrils than by the contamination the sight symbolized. The problem lay less with the smell of the rancid cesspool than with the sensitivity of the refined observer.

This trouble can be contextualized within the grander narratives of class and race and the expectations engendered by them. The English traveler, his mind perceiving the smells around him and registering them against the romanticized fragrances of his English childhood and against his presumptions about how Ireland would smell, may well have been less smitten by the country's odor than were Thomas Moore or Lady Morgan, whose perception was no less colored, but in their cases by a nationalism replete with preconceptions of how a romanticized Ireland *should* smell. By the same token, the heap of precious manure while foul to the middle-class observer may have been fragrant to the peasant farmer: recall that what George Moore perceived as "a stink," the "inmates" of the cottage described as "a warm smell." Yet the same molecules were surging into both parties' nostrils, binding to the olfactory receptors of each. Only their perceptions were different. The extended historical moment this paper examines is one in which the English middle class – and its Irish equivalent in anxious imitation – had already developed a lowered level of olfactory tolerance that did not yet prevail in rural Ireland.

The untutored Irish peasant was not disgusted by the proximity of the pig and the cesspool because he had not yet learned that he should be. He was, however, about to be taught. And his indoctrination, brought about not at the hands of the distrusted colonizer, but of a rising Irish middle class scrambling to distance itself from the stench of its fellow-Irishman, was one of the more astonishing transformations in the belated embourgeoisement of Catholic Ireland.

Reordering the Register

That transformation in smell perception occurred in France, as Alain Corbin has detailed, more than a century earlier. Smells were, as never before, observed and noted; the thresholds of olfactory tolerance were abruptly lowered so that odors once unremarkable were now suspect. A new awareness of the putrid spread throughout the social body. As the wealthy de-odorized themselves it was from the poor that stinks were now detected. Smell became a weapon in the social contest. The fierce resistance with which the endeavor was met is evidenced by the struggles of municipal officials and sanitary reformers. Theirs was a "battle," Corbin reports, "against dung, filth, and vitiated air"; their enemy, the peasants' "loyalty to an *ancien régime* of sensory values" (1986: 211).

The Irish trajectory was no less contentious. The Parliamentary Act of 1854 targeting such "nuisances" as public cesspools and rotting animal corpses had little effect; public representatives remained "uninterested in change," often "actively hostile" to the sanitation laws (Robins 1995: 239). Prosecutions were few, government officials complaining "time and again" about the wholesale disregard for their regulations (Breathnach 2005: 126). Yet the awareness of stink was increasing. By the 1880s the middle-class child Stephen Dedalus, James Joyce's alter ego, knew the characteristic odor of the unfragrant peasant "at the back of the chapel at Sunday Mass ... a smell of air and rain and turf and corduroy" ([1916] 2007: 15). Dublin newspapers like *The Freeman's Journal* grumbled that the dungheap remained "an indispensable adjunct to the Irish peasant life" (January 22, 1887). But much of the peasantry remained unmoved: new registers of smell, they understood, signaled new systems of control. What was to be done? Enter the priest: "a king," wrote the French traveler Paul Dubois in 1908, "in his kingdom" (1908: 494). Trusted, revered, and feared, only he could tell the people that they stank.

The priest's authority was powerful but recent. The Catholic hierarchy had instigated in mid-century a transformation in the Irish Church so deep that scholars, following Emmet Larkin, now call it a "devotional revolution."[12] The project's determination to eradicate the disorderly remnants of semi-pagan beliefs and replace them with modern, authorized, disciplined practices applied as readily to home as to chapel. The operative term here is "replace," for the Catholic hierarchy's "civilizing mission" constituted not just a radical overhaul but a substitution of public and domestic practices in which purity of soul and cleanliness of the home became mutually authorizing public and private goods in the service of God – or at least of the institutional Church (Inglis 1998).

A realignment of olfactory references fell naturally within the remit of the devotional revolution, for instrumental in its astonishing success was an appeal to sensory perception. As the Church dismantled or regulated traditional rites of piety, it opened up the senses, as if in compensation, to novel experience. Ceremonies of grand theatricality were imported in which "the whole world of the senses was explored through music, singing, candles, vestments, and incense" (Larkin 1972: 645). Religious rituals, previously performed in the scattered homes of the faithful, were centralized in the new parish churches, designated spaces marked off from the secular world by the uplifting odors of chrism, beeswax, and smoldering frankincense. The odor of sanctity, one might say, displaced the stench of cowdung.

A transformation of the everyday, the devotional revolution introduced a new sense of sin, a "sensual Puritanism," that reconfigured what was decent and respectable, pleasurable and permissible (Larkin 1972: 645). As with devotional practices, sensory inputs were redefined as tolerable and illicit. Odors once thought acceptable, even agreeable, were now to be considered, by reframing within the discourses of ill-health, progress, and above all, morality, repugnant. As a result, the collective imagination of the Irish peasant was to be reshaped to induce in him revulsion to what he had hitherto found pleasing, and desire for a new series of olfactory experiences. His notion of disgust was to be reformulated in conformity with a modern, a European, most immediately an English, system of olfactory values. If reluctant, then he must first be made aware, then ashamed of, his primitive conditions. In the reconfiguration of the Gaelo-Catholic conscience, dirt was now to be indexed under the increasingly capacious category of sin, and shame, ever-present in the economy of Catholic social control, was to be mobilized to enforce the new order. Many young clergymen had come to know shame well.

It was common that immediately following ordination the newly-ordained Irish priest be deployed in one of the great cities of England.[13] Serving alongside the genteel clergy of England he was exposed, like Canon Patrick Sheehan's priestly hero, Luke Delmege, to a bourgeois regime of sensory perception. Visiting the foul Irish ghettoes he recognized that his fellow exiles lived, indeed, much as Engels had reported. He was the butt of anti-Irish prejudice. "Every man that lives amongst [the English] knows that they are always making jokes about Paddy and the pig" wrote another exile of the time, Michael Collins (qtd. in Garvin 1988: 55). The effect of these experiences, a contending mélange of admiration and shame that induced an inevitable *ressentiment*, propelled the clergyman's zeal for change on his return.[14]

Such a one was Fr Joseph Guinan, in whose many popular novels we can trace the shifting olfactory perceptions that underlay the transformation in Irish rural life. When Fr Devoy, of his *The Island Parish* (1908) returns to the land he had once thought fragrant all had seemingly changed. As if through new eyes he sees the marks of his people's degradation, "their slovenly, slatternly ways, their dirty houses, dirty clothes, dirty children" (Guinan 1908: 90). The taunt "dirty Irish" had been thrown time and again at him in England; now, he has to concede, there was "some foundation for the galling jibe" (ibid.: 82). He recalls the epithet with an anger intensified by shame. Like his creator, Fr Guinan, on his own return from Liverpool in 1900, the fictional priest determines to transform his parishioners. He will "educat[e] them into cultivating," not only "habits of tidiness and orderliness," but "a higher standard of taste" (ibid.: 90). "Sanitas Sanitatis" will be his battle cry (Guinan 1908: 82). He will institute "a crusade against dirt and unsanitary conditions" (ibid.: 82).

The home, bosom of the now mandated nuclear family was the target of the priest and the Church he represented. In the 1883 pages of *The Irish Ecclesiastical Record*, the "in-house" journal of the clergy, they had read salutary treatises on the terrors of air-borne disease. A series of articles entitled 'Sanitary Sermons' warned that contagion "floats in the air, it is stored up in the earth, and … may yet retain its vigour; it may be inhaled with the breath… It attacks man, and the brute creation; and spares neither palace nor cottage" (Cox (1883): 684). New cottages were required, each, like the priest himself, a beacon of civility, a model for emulation which

> should serve as a school of sanitation from which knowledge
> of the laws of health should spread in ever widening circles,
> until cleanliness should take the place of squalor, and Ireland
> could no longer be pointed at as the *enfant sale*. (ibid.)

Again, the exemplary priest provided the model, for the promise of this modern domesticity shone forth from his own genteel arrangements. "A cosey nest indeed," remarked Canon Sheehan's Fr Dan on entering his young curate's abode, where "the fire burnt merrily … cleanliness, neatness, tidiness, taste everywhere; the etchings and engravings gave tone to the walls; the piano lay open, as if saying "come touch me"; the books…" he sighs … "altogether … a picture of delight" (1900: 57). A bourgeois idyll, a rural Irish incarnation of the "House Beautiful," it was a catalogue of middle-class orderliness and sensory delights; it could hardly be more unlike the rank Irish cabin.[15]

Women were the key to this transformation. The kitchen would become the space in which her new identity as "housewife" would be forged, the "cloister," thought Fr William Lockington SJ, "wherein she reigns as queen" (1921: 111). "Modest, retiring, home-keeping, kindly and gentle," the keeper of the Irish home, advised Guinan, could, "like Mary," be "the Mistress of the Holy House" (1908: 112). Under such direction, Tom Inglis confirms, women "transform[ed] the confined space in which they operated from what was in reality an animal house to a modern, civilized home" (1998: 197). And as those cabins made way for modern cottages, "the primitive and uncleanly habits" of the people that Fr Devoy had decreed intolerable became, indeed, less tolerated (Guinan 1908: 151). In their place were installed new internal and external practices, ordained to be carried out with near-religious devotion by the woman of the house, authorized by the Immaculate Queen of Heaven by whose writ she cleaned the bodies and preserved the souls of her charges.

If the Church's new domestic ideology had unveiled in the spotless mother the aspirational model of Irish womanhood, so the determinedly single male was frequently presented as its sinful counter-type to be shamed and ridiculed. The "old bachelors of the parish" ("and their name was legion"), Guinan grumbles, were incorrigible (1908: 151). Missionary priests, the shock troops of the devotional revolution whose purpose it was "to heighten, in a cumulative way the penitent's consciousness of sin," came to badger the old men in sermons (Prost, Larkin, and Freudenberger 1998: 12). "Again and again," writes Guinan, the preachers referred "in scathing terms, to [the bachelors'] miserable, forlorn condition, unsanitary houses, selfishness, cowardice, and spiritual destitution generally" (1908: 151). Surrounded by their pigs, untroubled by the putridity, they sought refuge in a reassuring past. Their literary incarnation is the Old-Grey-Fellow, comic villain of *The Poor Mouth*.[16]

A repository of ancient proverb, shibboleth, and blarney masquerading as wisdom, the Old Fellow is, in Declan Kiberd's phrase, "the stage Gael," a Gaelically-masked reiteration of the stage Irishman himself (1996: 502). A mockery of Irish manliness, this vainglorious layabout recognizes in the sweeping brush of the woman, mark of freedom for her, the instrument of his future subordination. In a desperate reassertion of patriarchal authority he makes one final appeal to tradition.

At the end of yet another day boiling potatoes for Ambrose and sweeping once more his detritus from her house the Old-Grey-Fellow charges the mother with Ungaelicism. Untrue to her destiny, she had refused to bend to the "*cinniúint Ghaelach*," her traditional Gaelic fate. Bring it all back in, woman, the Old Fellow commands.

"And," the narrator tells us, "she did so."

She took a bucket full of muck, mud and ashes and hen's droppings from the roadside and spread it around the hearth gladly in front of me. When everything was arranged, I moved over near the fire and for five hours I became a child in the ashes – a raw youngster rising up according to the old Gaelic tradition. Later at midnight I was taken and put into bed, but the foul stench of the fireplace stayed with me for a week; it was a stale, putrid smell and I do not think that the like will ever be there again. (O'Brien [1941] 1993: 16)

The like of that stench, and the Irishness it had come to represent, would indeed never be in the Irish cottage again. The desperate attempt by the Old-Grey-Fellow to keep the pig in his parlor, to hold, that is, to a system of values antecedent to embourgeoisement and to make of his native dirt a *cordon sanitaire culturel* that would keep modernity at bay, would come to naught.

The woman of the house had dared to sweep from the whitewashed cottage, as the modern world was sweeping from Ireland, the odors of a Gaelic past once perceived as reassuring, now coded as offensive, even morally suspect. And if she and the new social order of modern hygiene she embodied had been thwarted by a model of Irish masculinity that clung anxiously to the remnants of a doomed past, it would not be for long. Despite the recalcitrance of the Irish peasant – now exposed by O'Brien as the obtuseness of the reactionary male – the new order of domesticity did come to reign over the cottages of Ireland. Though much was lost along this path to modernity, it was in large part a liberating dispensation and it was enabled by an entente of Irish priest and Irish mother. Together they would transform hovels into homes and reconstruct the smellscape of Ireland.

Acknowledgments

I would like to thank my colleagues for reading earlier drafts of this essay: Kevin Kenny, Vera Kreilkamp, James M.Smith, and Christopher Wilson.

Notes

1. First published in Irish in 1941 as *An Béal Bocht*, the novel is undeservedly neglected in English language criticism. See, however, Clissman (1975), Kiberd (2001), McKibben (2003) on gender in the novel. Also, see Clune and Hurson (1997), Cronin ([1989] 1998), Shea (1992), Hopper (1995), and (in Irish) Ó Conaire (1986). Patrick C. Power's masterly 1964 English translation is enhanced in the Dalkey Archive 1996 edition by Ralph Steadman's illustrations.
2. Thanks to Vera Kreilkamp and Perry Curtis for drawing my attention to this extract.
3. While some of the artworks Kinmonth has assembled present clearly romanticized views of rural Ireland, many of the artists, particularly engravers for illustrated magazines unhampered by artistic illusions, seem determined on verisimilitude.
4. See Bakhtin [1930] 1981, Corbin (1986), Fabre-Vassas (1997), Malcomson and Mastoris (1998), and Stallybrass and White (1986). On disgust, see Darwin (1872); in modern theories of

emotion, see Rozin, Haidt, and McCauley (1993); for a contrary view on the social nature of disgust see Miller (1998, 2005).

5. James Joyce most memorably employed the fact as metaphor describing Ireland as "the old sow that eats her farrow" ([1916] 2007: 147).

6. While what a particular facial expression tells us varies from culture to culture, Ekman believes that the evidence for disgust having a universal facial expression is strongest (along with happiness, sadness, anger, and fear/surprise) (1999).

7. Haidt's classification of disgust as a "basic" emotion is not quite universally accepted; indeed, the designation "basic," is itself contested (Ekman 1999).

8. We share with Darwin the intuitive belief that facial expressions are the outward manifestations of emotions within. We smile *because* we are happy. But emotions may not be the answer to why we do things. The standard "natural kind" model of emotion that provides a scientific warrant for our commonsense approach has recently been questioned. Emotions, Lisa Feldman Barrett contends, do not "carve nature at its joints" (2006: 45). Anger, fear, disgust, for example, do not "refer to the things being classified, but rather are classification schemes that people impose on the world during perception" (ibid.: 46).

9. I do not use the phrase "threat of ejection" metaphorically. Deportation of Irish paupers was legal despite the island's integration. Official reports by the Massachusetts Commissioners of Alien Passengers and Foreign Paupers confirm that forcible ejections were also carried out in the United States. (My thanks to Hide Hirota for bringing these cases to my attention.)

10. "Soft" as distinct from the acrid smell of coal with which urban middle-class houses were heated.

11. This enables pigs to survive well on human waste. Miller (1990) estimates that with Chinese breeds (imported to Ireland from mid-century onwards) four young pigs could derive sustenance from the excrement of a family of four humans. Potato consumption in mid-nineteenth-century Ireland was "astronomical" – between eight and fourteen pounds per adult per day (Davies 1994: 557). A consumption to elimination ratio of 5:1 suggests two to three pounds of human waste excreted per person per day.

12. Attendance at religious ceremonies is one measure of its success. Weekly mass-going rose from around 30 to 40 percent in rural Ireland in the 1840s to about 90 percent or more by the end of the century.

13. Accurate figures are difficult to come by. Brophy suggests that one-third of all Irish clergymen spent some time abroad immediately after ordination.

14. Identification with the admired colonizer was always a danger: after two years in London, even the fiercely nationalist Canon Sheehan had "discard[ed] the rich brogue of his mother tongue,

so welcome to the Irish ear," reports his sympathetic biographer (Heuser 1917: 75). He had become, in a term Guinan borrowed from his parishioners, "Inglified."

15. While my emphasis is on the role of the Catholic clergy, others such as Ó Gráda (1977) and MacPherson (2001) have illustrated how central were the Irish co-operative movement and the journal *The Irish Homestead* in the production of domesticity.

16. The novel's chief delight, perhaps, lies in its upending of the pieties that surrounded the island autobiography *An tOileánach* by Tomás Ó Crohan (Tomás Ó Criomhthain). This text, known mostly in translation, was revered in patriotic circles for its depiction of a simpler, nobler way of Gaelic life. At one point Ó Crohan remarks that in the island houses two beds were typical, under one of which would be a couple of pigs, and under the other potatoes: *Bhíodh dhá mhuic ag dul fé leabaidh acu agus bhíodh prátaí fén gceann eile* ([1929] 2002: 331). Robin Flower's English translation of 1934, however, overlooks the pigs claiming only that "Potatoes would be stored under these beds" – an omission all the more remarkable for "the cow or two, calf or two, the ass [and] the dog" he felt it unnecessary to banish from the living quarters (Ó Crohan [1934] 1978: 27). To the Irish parlor evidently, anything bar pigs could be admitted. My thanks to Brendan Kane for drawing my attention to this and the many other instances of pig-elision in the translated text.

References

Bakhtin, Mikhail. [1930] 1981. *The Dialogical Imagination: Four Essays*. Austin, TX: University of Texas.

Barrett, Lisa F. 2006. "Are Emotions Natural Kinds?" *Perspectives on Psychological Science* 1, 28–58.

Bourke, Joanna. 1993. *Husbandry to Housewifery: Women, Economic Change, and Housework in Ireland, 1890–1914*. Oxford: Clarendon Press.

Bourke, Joanna. 1999. "The Ideal Man: Irish Masculinity and the Home, 1880–1914." In Marilyn Cohen and Nancy Curtin (eds), *Reclaiming Gender: Transgressive Identities in Modern Ireland*. New York: St Martin's Press.

Bourke, P.M.A. 1965. The Agricultural Statistics of the 1841 Census of Ireland. A Critical Review. *The Economic History Review*, 18, 376–91.

Bourke, P.M.A. 1993. *The Visitation of God? The Potato and the Great Irish Famine*. Dublin: Liliput Press.

Breathnach, Ciara. 2005. *The Congested Districts Board of Ireland, 1891–192: Poverty and Development in the West of Ireland*. Dublin, Ireland; Portland, OR: Four Courts Press.

Carleton, William. [1847] 1979. *Traits and Stories of the Irish Peasantry, Second Series*. New York: Garland Pub.

Carlyle, Thomas. 1882. *Reminiscences of My Irish Journey, 1849*. London: Sampson Low, Marston, Searle & Rivington.

Clissman, Anne. 1975. *Flann O'Brien: A Critical Introduction to His Writings*. Dublin: Gill and Macmillan.

Clune, Anne and Hurson, Tess (eds) 1997. *Conjuring Complexities: Essays on Flann O'Brien*. Dublin: The Institute of Irish Studies.

Commonwealth, T. S. O. T. 1858–60. Report of the Commissioners of Alien Passengers and Foreign Paupers. Boston, MA: William White, Printer to the State.

Corbin, Alain. 1986. *The Foul and the Fragrant: Odor and the French Social Imagination*, Cambridge, MA: Harvard University Press.

Cox, Michael F. 1883. 'Sanitary Sermons,' *Irish Ecclesiastical Record*, November (4): 684.

Curtis, L.P. 1968. *Anglo-Saxons and Celts: A Study of Anti-Irish Prejudice in Victorian England*. New York: New York University Press.

Curtis, L.P. [1971] 1997. *Apes and Angels*. Washington, DC: Smithsonian Institute Press.

Cronin, Anthony. 1998. *No Laughing Matter: The Life and Times of Flann O'Brien*. New York: Fromm International Pub.

Darwin, Charles. [1872] 1979. *The Expression of Emotions in Man and Animals*. London, New York: Julian Friedmann; St. Martin's Press.

Davies, J.E. 1994. "Giffen Goods, the Survival Imperative, and the Irish Potato Culture." *The Journal of Political Economy*, 102: 547–65.

Dubois, Paul. 1908. *Contemporary Ireland (L'Irlande Contemporaine)*. Dublin: Maunsel & Co.

Ekman, Paul. 1999. "Basic Emotions." In Tim Dalgleish and Michael J. Power (eds), *Handbook of Cognition and Emotion*. New York: Wiley & Sons.

Engels, F. [1845] 1942. *The Condition of the Working Class in England in 1844*. London: George Allen & Unwin Ltd.

Fabre-Vassas, Claudine. 1997. *The Singular Beast: Jews, Christians and the Pig*. New York: Columbia University Press.

Ferris, Ina. 2002. *The Romantic National Tale and the Question of Ireland*. Cambridge: Cambridge University Press.

Garvin, Tom. 1988. *Nationalist Revolutionaries in Ireland, 1858–1928*. Oxford, New York: Clarendon Press, Oxford University Press.

Guinan, James. 1908. *The Island Parish*. Dublin Waterford: M. H. Gill & Son Ltd.

Hall, S.C. 1883. *Retrospect of a Long Life*. London: R. Bentley & Sons.

Heuser, Herman. J. 1917. *Canon Sheehan of Doneraile: The Story of an Irish Parish Priest as Told Chiefly by Himself in Books, Personal Memoirs and Letters*. New York: Longmans Green and Co.

Hopper, Keith. 1995. *Flann O'Brien: A Portrait of the Artist as a Young Post-Modernist*. Cork: Cork University Press.

Inglis, Tom. 1998. *Moral Monopoly: The Rise and Fall of the Catholic Church in Modern Ireland*. Dublin: University College Dublin Press.

Joyce, James. [1916] 2007. *A Portrait of the Artist as a Young Man*. New York: Norton & Co.

Kennedy, Brian. P. 1993. "The Traditional Irish Thatched House: Imagery and Reality, 1793–1993." In Adele Dalsimer (ed.), *Visualizing Ireland: National Identity and the Pictorial Tradition*. Boston, MA: Faber and Faber.

Kiberd, Declan. 1996. *Inventing Ireland*. London: Random House.

Kinmonth, Claudia. 2006. *Irish Rural Interiors in Art*. New Haven, CT; London: Yale University Press.

Larkin, Emmet. J. 1972. "The Devotional Revolution in Ireland, 1850–75." *The American Historical Review, 77*: 625–52.

Lee, J.J. 1973. *The Modernisation of Irish Society, 1848–1918*. Dublin: Gill and Macmillan.

Lockington, William J. 1921. *The Soul of Ireland*. New York: The Macmillan Company.

McKibben, Sarah. 2003. "*The Poor Mouth*: A Parody of (Post) Colonial Irish Manhood." *Research in African Literatures*, 34: 96–114.

MacPherson, James. 2001. "'Ireland Begins in the Home': Women, Irish National Identity, and the Domestic Sphere in *The Irish Homestead*, 1896–1912." *Éire–Ireland*, 36: 131–52.

Malcolmson, Robert and Stephanos Mastoris. 1998. *The English Pig: A History*. London: Hambledon

Miller, Robert. L. 1990. "Hogs and Hygiene." *The Journal of Egyptian Archaeology*, 76: 125–40.

Miller, William Ian. 1998. *The Anatomy of Disgust*. Cambridge, MA: Harvard University Press.

Miller, William Ian. 2005. "Darwin's Disgust." In David Howes (ed.), *Empire of the Senses*. New York: Berg.

Moore, George. [1886] 2004. *Parnell and His Island*. Dublin: University College Dublin Press.

Newcomer, James. 1967. *Maria Edgeworth the Novelist: 1767–1849, a Bicentennial Study*. Fort Worth, TX: Christian University Press.

O'Brien, Flann. 1993. *An Béal Bocht; The Poor Mouth: A Bad Story About the Hard Life*. London: Flamingo.

O'Brien, Flann. [1967] 1999. *The Third Policeman*. Dublin: Dalkey Archive Press.

Ó Conaire, Breandán. 1986. *Myles Na Gaeilge: Lámhleabhar Ar Shaothar Ghaeilge Bhrian Ó Nualláin*. Dublin: An Clóchomhar Tta.

Ó Crohan, (Ó Criomhthain) Tomás. [1934] 1978. *The Islandman*. Translated by Robin Flower. Oxford: Oxford University Press.

Ó Crohan, (Ó Criomthain) Tomás. [1929] 2002. *An tOileánach*. Dublin: Cló Talbóid.

Ó Gráda, Cormac. 1977. "The Beginnings of the Irish Creamery System, 1880–1914." *The Economic History Review*, 30: 284–305.

Owenson, Sidney. (Lady Morgan). 1850. *The Wild Irish Girl*. London, Henry Colburn.

Porteus, J. Douglas. "Smellscape." In Jim Drobnick (ed.), *The Smell Culture Reader*. New York: Berg.

Prost, J., Larkin, E.J., and Freudenberger, H. 1998. *A Redemptorist Missionary in Ireland, 1851–1854: Memoirs by Joseph Prost*. Cork: Cork University Press.

Robins, Joseph. 1995. *The Miasma: Epidemic and Panic in Nineteenth-Century Ireland*. Dublin: Institute of Public Administration.

Rozin, P., Haidt, J., and McCauley, C.R. 1993. "Disgust." In Michael Lewis and Jeanette M. Haviland (eds), *Handbook of Emotions*. New York: The Guildford Press.

Shea, Thomas F. 1992. *Flann O'Brien's Exorbitant Novels*. Lewisburg, PA: Bucknell University Press.

Sheehan, Patrick. A. 1900. *My New Curate; a Story Gathered from the Stray Leaves of an Old Diary*. Boston, MA: Marlier & Co.

Sheehan, Patrick. A. 1901. *Luke Delmege*. New York: Longmans Green and Co.

Stallybrass, Peter and White, Allon. 1986. *The Politics and Poetics of Transgression*. Ithaca, NY: Cornell University Press.

Weimer, Martin. 1993. *Das Bild der Iren und Irlands im Punch 1841–1921*. Frankfurt: Peter Lang.

Wills, Clair. 2001. "Women, Domesticity and the Family: Recent Feminist Work in Irish Cultural Studies." *Cultural Studies*, 15: 33–57.

Senses & Society | VOLUME 4, ISSUE 3
PP 303–322 | REPRINTS AVAILABLE DIRECTLY FROM THE PUBLISHERS | PHOTOCOPYING PERMITTED BY LICENSE ONLY

Fearless Trembling: A Leap of Faith into the Devil's Frying Pan

Patrick Laviolette

Patrick Laviolette teaches in the School of Visual & Material Culture at Massey University where he is Director of Postgraduate Studies. He has published a dozen journal articles and presented 45 papers in 15 different countries. This piece is an extended précis of his forthcoming book, 'Not a Hap-Hazardous Sport'.
p.laviolette@massey.ac.nz

ABSTRACT   Phenomenologically and reflexively influenced, this paper investigates an experiential conception of the imagination through an exploration of an extreme bodily act. Foremost, it sets the scene for a conceptual consideration of dangerous practices such as cliff jumping. This potentially pushes the level in which we can reflect upon such a thing as an existential or embodied imagination. Here modernity's leveling of the docile body is challenged. Hence, in focusing on those sub-cultural practices that involve the extreme use of landscape, I propose an alternative scenario in which to consider the creativity of the body. Such a framework situates hazardous activities beyond the level of much contemporary thinking within the anthropology of sport or the sociology of risk, to a more far-reaching – perhaps "extremist" position – where they come

DOI 10.2752/174589209X12464528171897

**across as existentially poignant, performative acts
of the social imagination.**

KEYWORDS: embodied imagination, cliff jumping, extreme
landscapes, existential anthropology

long live the dance in the whirl of the infinite;
long live the wave that hides me in the abyss;
long live the wave that hurls me up above the stars.

(Kierkegaard [1843] 1983)

This passage by Søren Kierkegaard provides an apt introduction to a paper on the relationship between the imagination and extreme acts such as cliff jumping, especially since it is taken from his book *Fear and Trembling*. Fitting because the sensations of fear and trembling are important parts of the experience of staring down at the waves that crash against the rocks while contemplating, from high above the cliff face, the idea of leaping into the sea. But this is a different type of "landscape of fear" to that which the geographer Yi-Fu Tuan had in mind in his volume of the same name. Rather, it is one where his concept of "topophilia" – of a deep empathy with the environment – equally applies (1980; 1974).

The notion of fear and trembling that I consider here is therefore part of a sensuous reflexivity. As the present article reveals, the ethnographic game can indeed be taken to several extremes. These not only involve imaginary and genuine risks for informants and researchers alike, but, equally, an existential challenge to the notion of performance, the nature of the imagination and even the character of ethnographic research. Hence, through the practice of cliff jumping in Cornwall UK, this paper explores the conceptual link between a prospective anthropology of the imagination and a reflexively based existential phenomenology (Jackson 2005; Karl and Hamalian [1963] 1973; Tilley 1994). In reflecting upon an embodied imagination, I suggest that engaging with the very practices of research in the social sciences, in all their forms, is in itself part of taking a figurative – and as this article demonstrates – sometimes also a literal "leap of faith."

The Devil's Frying-Pan is a locally famous cove in Cornwall where young people engage with such leaps on a regular basis. This site is owned by the National Trust and is located near the village of Cadgwith on the east side of the most southern tip of the Lizard peninsula. For my informants in the village of Mullion, roughly 6 miles away, it is perhaps the quintessential cliff jump in the area, to which most new-coming practitioners are eventually introduced once they have gained a bit of experience and developed a certain bravado from easier jumps. "Trust me, ya need to build up to this one. It's not called the Devil's Frying-Pan for nothing," states Ally (aged twenty-seven), who boasts having made the jump twice in her "youth" but would not dream of doing it again now. She continues,

> I think it gets its name from the actual shape of the cove and the way the water actually swells up and bubbles like oil in a frying-pan … that's the worst part of this jump 'cause even if it's a safeish jump, it's still a really eerie and sinister kinda place, no fooling.

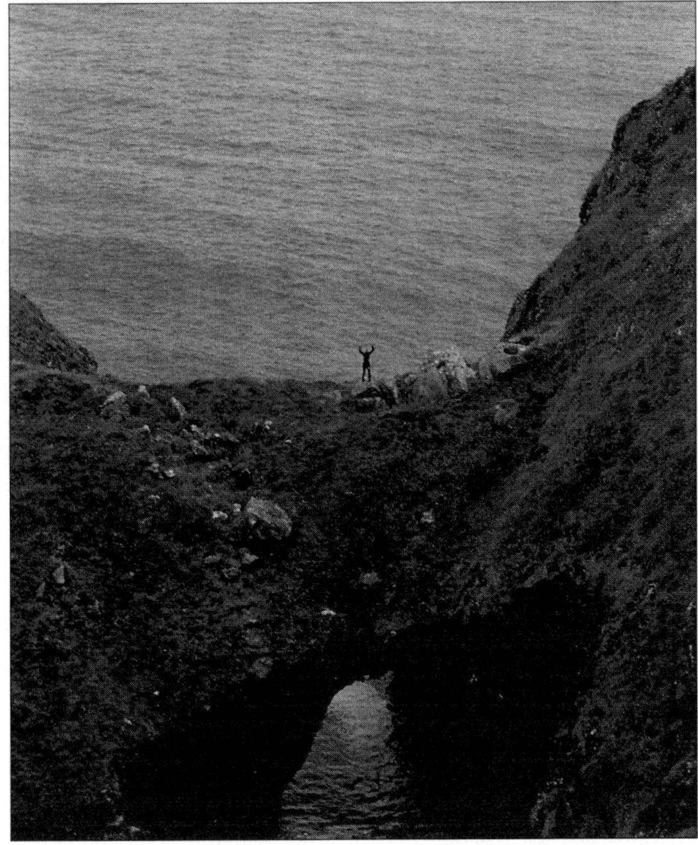

Figure 1
The Devil's Frying-Pan, Cadgwith, Lizard Peninsula.

My first face-to-face encounter with the Devil's Frying-Pan really was a leap of faith on many levels. Firstly, because it was a complete ordeal just to rally the enthusiasm to be taken by my friends. It was like pulling teeth. In May of 2003, I had tried to convince the "Mullion Crew" to take me to the Frying-Pan but they were simply not interested. They kept saying I was too old to be engaging in these types of crazy teenager activities. "The advantage of reaching your thirties is that you don't have to do stupid things like that anymore … you clearly don't want to get any older do you? Mid-life crisis already old boy?" These were the types of comments that Ally's partner Mike kept making.

So I never made it that time, but I was determined to go during a later visit at the end of July 2003. Upon leaving the pub one night, I thought I had convinced Mike to go on Thursday afternoon, after his work. I rang him after lunch and got more banter about being insane. He then said that he had scheduled a band rehearsal. I was beginning to think that this Devil's Frying-Pan thing was cursed. But somehow I eventually convinced him to go the following day. Five of us – plus baby and dog in tow – set off from Mullion on Friday at midday. They were Ally, Mike, and their dog with their friends Ron, Julie, and their daughter Coral (who is the only person in this article not to appear under a pseudonym).

The Pan would not give up its secrets that easily, however. This notorious jump also became a leap of faith because once we arrived, we had considerable problems in physically accessing the site. There was overgrowth of gorse, nettles, and thorns all around. It was sheer determination and even obsessiveness which allowed me to reach it, driven by my conviction that I had to do this jump and protected by a wetsuit which allowed me to pile through the otherwise impenetrable thicket of bushes. The Frying-Pan seems to be such an important and symbolic jump partly because of its many barriers. Conquering the physical obstacles made the experience quite significant in my own limited biography of jumping. But the barriers were also social. Indeed, not being easily put off by the reticence of my informants was important. It is worth noting that all of them stipulated that the site had changed considerably over the past decade since they were last there, perhaps, one of them even suggested, as a National Trust deterrent to the practice of cliff jumping.

Not only was this jump a leap of faith for me because the others were themselves not prepared to participate but also because, given the difficulty of access, they were not even able to spectate either. In fact, no one saw me jump. So one has to take it on good faith that I actually did. Though if you ask any of my four companions, I am sure that there is no doubt in their minds to the contrary. For one thing, they would testify, as they did to me, that they clearly heard the incredibly loud splashes when I hit the water. Given that I was upwind from them, they also explained how they distinctly heard my screams of terror, particularly on my second jump, which I felt I should mark out by yelling something. Since I could not think of anything clever I simply shouted, leaving them slightly worried, especially when I did not hear, and thus did not reply to, their inquiries as to my well being. My point here is that even though they never saw my jumps, the other senses have provided indications of the validity of my claim.

Given that there was no one present to witness this jump or capture it on film, I was clearly doing it as a challenge to myself – for the pure experience factor. This was highlighted to me by Ron once we arrived on site. He jested that it was surely enough that I had now seen the place and had taken some photos: "So you don't actually have to go through with it, we won't tell anyone, no one will know the difference right? Let's go then." He was of course been facetious. But he was also touching on the importance that I needed to overcome the access barriers if I really wanted to understand what this was all about. The gauntlet was down.

Similarly, the jump was again a leap of faith because my friends were not immediately present to reassure me, and be reassured, that everything was going well. Nor were they able to encourage me or share any strategic information about the site. Not having anyone there to "spot me," jumping blind as it were, was rather stressful. Hence it was much more part of an existential rather than an un-reflexive experience. There is a definite feeling that more things can go wrong when jumping alone, but also that it is a more individualistic, even liminal, moment. In a sense, then, even if it was not my initiation into jumping, I nonetheless felt that this was a type of ritual process.

In the end, all my jumps lasted a few seconds in total, a quarter of an hour with the climbing. Nevertheless, the event itself lasted several hours. It is worth noting that this type of solo jumping means nobody is there to share the actual experience with you on the day. Consequently, I could not find out from anyone else other than myself what the experience was like *in situ*. Ethnographically this is a strange turn of events. I was participating in something in which my inform-ants were not. But actually this did not matter so much because I now had their "respect," and had potentially achieved a level of embodied empathy. I had done something that was once a significant part of their lives. And, maybe more importantly, the afternoon's jumping provided a good means of accessing certain social memories as well as soliciting loads of jumping stories afterwards. The vignette above demonstrates certain methodological aspects in studying cliff jumping from a phenomenological perspective. You can always contrive a situation to talk with and interview people about this activity, but it is not until it becomes a natural topic of conversation based on the day's events that you really arrive at a level of understanding of how the imagination exists in and through this fleeting embodied experience (Hunter and Csikszentmihalyi 2000).

Sensuous Leisure

Cornwall is the most south-westerly peninsula of mainland Britain. With over 240 miles of coastline, tourism, fishing, and other seaside activities are central to this territory's socioeconomic identities (Busby and Laviolette 2006; Ireland 1989). Despite a rich and diverse social history – which are sources of distinction for many – this constituency is still one of Europe's poorest, having received European Objective 1 level funding in 1999. To an extent, this economic impoverishment results from the area's rapid de-industrialization, sociopolitical marginality, and dependence on a fluctuating and seasonal tourist trade. Perceptions thus clash as to whether Cornwall exists as a land apart or as a quintessentially British periphery.

It is not unusual for people to appropriate marginalized landmarks by personifying them with vernacular names and therefore associating them with their own particular causes. This gives special relevance to a site and the issue. By ascribing their own experiences to such locales, they are projecting onto them a stylized sense of the region as they think it should be (Crang 1997). As Setha Low and Denise Lawrence-Zuniga (2003) remind us, place becomes an agent, an embodied surrogate for values, desires, and dreams. The imagination is a crucial factor for understanding these processes. Yet it is still usually seen as images and dreams engendered in the mind through cognitive and cerebral processes. This article challenges such a conception, perhaps even turns it on its head in a way reminiscent of the recent work of Fernandez and Huber (2001). Thinking along these lines, the aim here is to emphasize the embodied nature of imaginative events.

Gaston Bachelard is an obvious point of reference for any concern with the anthropology of the imagination. Given the basis of the present research, as well as the phenomenological and reflexive caveat that I have outlined above, we particularly need to consider his groundbreaking exploration of the material imagination through his reflections on the elemental substances of fire, water, air, and earth ([1938] 1987; [1942] 1983; [1943] 1988; [1947] 1988). Indeed, Bachelard bears witness to the imaginative human freedom whereby we are asked to lay aside or suspend preconceptions. Instead we are encouraged to cultivate a capacity for awe and wonder. But he nonetheless falls into a Husserlian phenomenological perspective which prefaces the transcendence of our cognitive faculties (Husserl 1931). That is, Bachelard still views the originality of the poetic imagination as an opening up of ourselves to the revelations of the image as opposed to an opening up to experience. Or even more radically, where the image or experience would open up the potential for the imagination itself to be possible. Consequently, Bachelard suggests that our experience of the world does not guide our imagination but rather is guided by it.

Significant though his contributions are, and indeed heavily relied upon in what follows, I nevertheless want to open up some of these normative Bachelardian perspectives concerning the cognitive imagination. Conversely, I propose that the interaction of body, landscape, and danger is an experiential and existential arena in which the imagination can be acted out. The practice of stretching the mind and body to the limits – and of playing with life and death – establishes an ontological basis for an embodied creativity, for a creativity of the body.

Before addressing such theoretical issues explicitly, it is important to describe ethnographically the situation of cliff jumping in Cornwall. Also sometimes referred to as tombstoning, coasteering, and deep water soloing, cliff jumping is becoming increasingly popular as an extreme practice in Cornwall and in the UK generally. Although the activity is not unique to Cornwall most of my informants very strongly believe that it is enshrouded in the Cornish peninsula's own particular seaside and surf culture. In relation to the materiality of waves in the context of this aspect of Cornish culture, I have elsewhere examined the relationships between sewage and surfing, protest and pleasure (Laviolette 2006b).

Despite being among the most unregulated of extreme sports, cliff jumping now seems to be crossing over into a more formal and accepted public arena through competitions and corporate advertising. The basic premise is simple: to dive, or most often, jump feet first into the sea from as many different places and heights as possible. According to many avid enthusiasts, the Cornish coast provides an ideal scenario for jumping. It is scenic, with hundreds of isolated coves, bays, and steep rock faces that line a shore of relatively clean water, kept fairly warm by the area's characteristically mild and "Riviera-esque" climate (Thornton 1993). Equally important to them, this coastline is relatively accessible, both in its physical proximity as well as because it is not particularly residential or industrial – that is, not built up or overcrowded and access is not restricted.

As far as the social profile of those who jump is concerned, it ranges from those with a privileged upbringing to those from family backgrounds with much lower levels of economic, social, and cultural capital. As regards gender, I would estimate that even though women do figure less prominently than men, the ratio is more balanced than might be expected, perhaps 3:1. The most common inhibitory factor is age. Indeed, for some jumping starts when they are children (ten or twelve years of age) and drops dramatically after the teen years. In some cases people continue to jump into their thirties and forties, although this is less usual.

Part of the corporal significance of this activity is perhaps not so much that it permits an intense adrenaline rush as that it allows for the engagement and exploration of all the physical senses. Touch (to a great degree, but filtered through the wetsuit), sight, sound, smell, and the taste of salt water are all essential to the safe and successful enjoyment of the experience. Jumping is therefore in part about enhancing the potential for a full synesthetic experience, in which one can merge the sensation of free falling with an endearing encounter of body, air, land, and sea.

There is, therefore, an intermingling of our physical senses. More interestingly, however, it is not the phenomena of synesthesia as such that is most importantly at work here. Instead we should talk of some anomalous form of aesthesia – a combination or hybridisation of dysesthesia and kinesthesia. In other words, take into account the distortion, transformation, and acceleration of the senses rather than their blurring or blending (Bell and Lyall 2001). Indeed, particularly underwater, the experiences of touch, smell, taste, sound, and sight

Figure 2
Piskie Cove, Praa Sands.

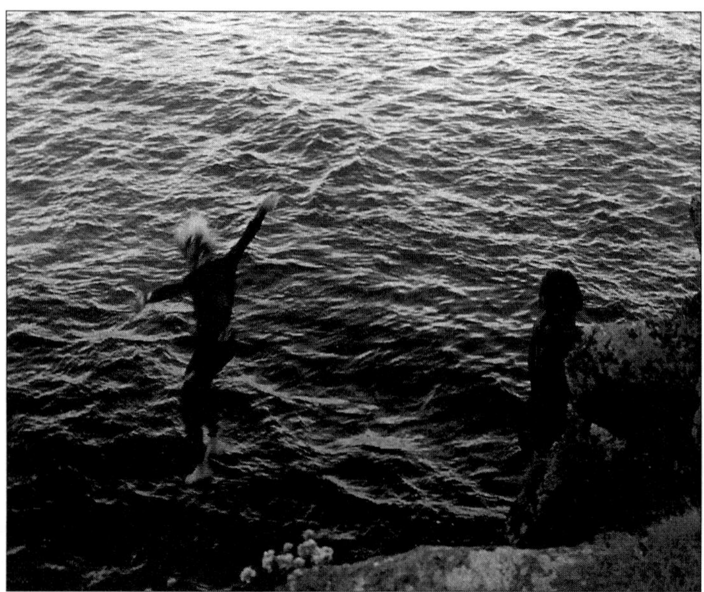

are not what we normally perceive them to be. Water as a medium actually alters our physical perceptions. It gives us a different type of experiential exposure. Furthermore, the activity of cliff jumping distorts our conventional notions of time and spatial perception. Events are rushed up or slowed in a disproportional way so that our sensation of time shifts temporarily. Schutz refers to this empathic and mimetic inversion of experience as a type of "reciprocity of perspectives" (1970: 183).

This sensorial confusion and overdrive is a significant justification put forward by many participants. Moreover, it is frequently this distorted modality of experience that is excessively sought by those participants who seek to engage in extreme sports during moments where they have altered their states of mind through drug or alcohol use (Lyng 1990). The words of one informant in his early forties sums up this "work hard play harder" ethos, commenting on his own lifestyle motto: "Contrary to popular belief I don't live on the edge, I live on the ledge over the edge".

One of the things used to distinguish cliff jumping from many other extreme practices is that this activity has a minimal reliance on equipment, especially safety gear. This is a significant factor in the relative lack of regulation of tombstoning in comparison to similar dangerous games: "cliff jumping is unique in that it's a mish-mash of many sports. At the end of the day though, I'd say it was most like sky diving with a big watery crash matt instead of a chute" states Rick (aged twenty-seven) from Porthleven. This minimal use of equipment demonstrates that jumping from cliffs is often about reducing restrictions and maximizing the potential for a fully embodied euphoria. As Rick claims, there's something quite primeval, primitive, even animalistic at work. Of course you have to have all your wits about you but really jumping is one of those acts where your instincts take over almost completely … it's about letting loose and relying on gut reactions.

A more radical seasoned jumper recounts,

I myself have been cliff jumping now for almost four years. My opinions vary to other jumpers as far as equipment goes. I am more the traditional jumper, wearing only a pair of shorts and a vest. This, I find, is much more natural and the pain is more intense.

Cliff jumpers have much difficulty in describing the feeling they get from this practice. They claim that it is beyond the sensation of most adrenaline rushes. In Sharky's words, "It's just a euphoric feeling when you're in mid-air, knowing there's no guaranteed safety mechanism to help you and no way back." Nonetheless, here is a passage from my field notes on the sensation of my first jump:

June 6, 2003

My thoughts on this first jump is that it feels quite unnatural. This is not a normal or regular thing to be experiencing or feeling. So it's an interesting juxtaposition to be having this "exploration of nature" element as a significant part of the experience and discourse when really this physical sensation is completely at odds with what one would actually find as natural. I've never fallen from such a height before. Even as a youngster I never jumped from the 10 meter diving board in our local pool. I would not describe cliff jumping as anything close to a near death experience and yet this type of free fall was one of the most unusual and unnatural sensations I've ever had. Perhaps this is because it was so contrived from the outset. I was studying cliff jumping months before ever actually doing it. Or perhaps this is because it was my first initiation to jumping. But I'm assuming at this stage that one would have to jump almost every day for quite some time before one felt it was a natural sensation. Free falling is not socially mundane. Surely most people don't experience this sensation with much frequency or on a regular basis.

My jumping mates began doubling the number of jumps that I was doing. I was trying to absorb it all, take it all in. Also, to be honest, I was rather bewildered by the whole thing. I started showing obvious reserve and even felt myself shaking somewhat even though it wasn't out of fear as such. More like I started over-analyzing things. Some water from our wetsuits had accumulated on the run up to the take off point and I

> started worrying that without shoes or booties like those that the others were wearing, I might slip on take off.

Maybe the reason I started worrying was that I had been introduced to cliff jumping through narratives about it. Stories like this one:

> There was this one time, on a big(ish) jump, where I slipped just before take off and so went hurtling, almost head-over-heels, downwards … I hit the water with almighty force; jamming my jaw, chipping a tooth and spraining almost every muscle in my back. That was the most frightening experience of my life, but even with many less dramatic near-death experiences like that; I'm not put off. People love to hear these stories and the feeling of success is too great for me to stop, even though I know I'm going to feel pain every time I pull on my wetsuit.

This passage by Dom (aged twenty-four) one of Rick's mates from Helston highlights a significant relationship between performance, pleasure, and pain. Indeed, if you knew him and read between the lines, you would realize that he means "girls love to hear these stories." An interesting facet of the physicality and embodiment of the Cornish coast is the relation of place to the body, risk, and sexuality. The extreme sports circles are very much related to the club, rave, and art scenes. During the 1960s and 1970s, St Ives artists generated numerous links between the human figure and the hazards or sexuality of the Cornish landscape. This has reinforced a hedonistic conception of leisure that especially marks the mood of the Cornish seaside as a place where adventure and reinvigoration as well as sexual promiscuity and fornication have become holiday sub-themes. Surfing hotspots like Fistral beach and the Watergate Bay in Newquay, or the nudist coves near Porthcurno and at St Austell's Carlyon Bay allow for these types of celebrations of the body, so that they have become synonymous with both risk and the *risqué*.

This is perhaps not all that surprising, especially when we consider that such relationships are reflected in a lot of the contemporary literature on bodily risk which is often related to the threats and dangers associated with certain sexual practices and behavior (Douglas 1992; Caplan 2000). Hence, John Fiske has produced a model of the beach that defines it as an ambivalent and unpredictable zone that encompasses "a physically anomalous category between land and sea … Nature/Culture" (1989: 44–5). As I have commented elsewhere, extreme sports provide an erstwhile poorly explored example about the relationships between the search for freedom, risk taking, the celebration of the body, and feelings of local pride and community (Laviolette 2007). The following quotation from Ben (aged twenty-six), from Harlyn, supports this when he describes this activity as not for the faint-at-heart, but if done "safely", not naively by some (mostly tourists), then there is no other feeling like it that I have encountered yet … I have heard stories of those who have ripped open their skin on entry… Maybe this is a myth set up by a group of mates to keep others away from what they like doing.

Cliff jumping is thus related at some level to a feeling of local identity and belonging. Participants are often very protective of jumping spots and the local knowledge associated with the practice. Cliff jumping also suggests that extreme sport enthusiasts are not bound to place in some static sense. Even if they might in reality regularly be returning to the same coves and shorelines these beach loiterers strongly associate such activities with freedom and movement. Additionally, they are playing in what the sociologist Tim Dant (1998) calls a transitory surf zone that emphasizes fluidity, change, danger, and ecstasy. Besides, the majority of these participants rarely restrict themselves to specific spots. They share a general feeling of wanderlust and hunt the coast for the best conditions or the least crowded beaches.

Most cliff jumpers therefore feel that they are part of the same euphoria-seeking subculture – similar to, but also very different from, that inhabited by skateboarders and BASE jumpers. As is the case with frozen waterfall climbers (Ferrell 2001), each community of jumpers has a lexicon of names given to specific places or those people who have jumped in a remarkable way. For example, we have Andy's Arse Flop, Lad Cove, Point X, Sharky's Echo, Dominic's Seal Squisher, Seagull Gully, the Beth Style Streaker, Piskies Cove, and so forth.

Hence, cliff jumping is significantly about creating sociality (Abramson and Laviolette 2007). One interesting aspect of this sociality and conviviality, which seems to push even further the level of danger involved, is when people jump together as pairs or even three or four at a time. The sharing of fun and fear, as well as the increased potential for collision with each other, reinforces the trust between cliff jumpers. Further, it binds them together in more than just a shared experience, it unites them through a socially constructed group narrative – a mutual experience that embodies the imagination – and where the imagination is embodied.

Disembodied Free Fall: Death and the Politics of Jumping

But what about the disembodied free fall of the imagination? The importance of the sea for Cornwall's economy is extensive. But the sea has also been the taker of life through the perils of fishing and ship wrecks. Further, it has been the vehicle by which emigration was made possible in the eighteenth and nineteenth centuries. Hundreds of boats carried thousands of people to Australia, California, Canada,

Figure 3
Group of quay-side jumpers, Newquay.

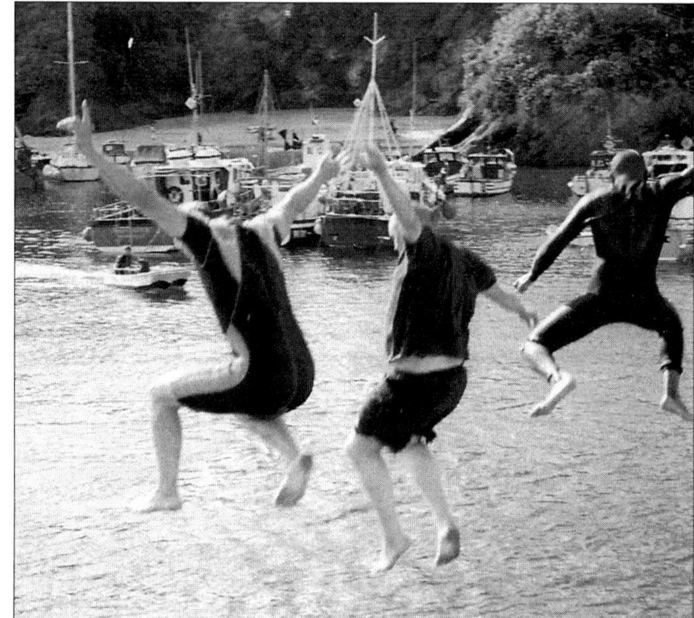

New Zealand, and South Africa. Cousin Jack and cousin Jane were taken away by the sea. Elsewhere I have discussed at more length the links between death and Cornish identity through the material metaphors concerning emigration, immigration, heritage tourism, and the hazards of Cornwall's industries (Laviolette 2003; 2006a). Indeed, the Cornish peninsula has often been seen as one informant states: "as a place where places end but never begin." Britishness, Englishness, and Cornishness reach their final destination in many of the duchy's places, no less at Land's End, the most western point of the "nation." As Alfred Tennyson says in his personal travel journal, "Funeral. Land's End and Life's End" (Tennyson, in 1949, quoted in Martin 1980: 320).

Given these linkages and my focus on existential anthropology, I want to elaborate on the associations between danger, death, and jumping. One informant I spoke to about cliff jumping told me that at least one death per year is caused by the sport. He said it was the most hazardous activity practiced by the young people in the region. Indeed, on June 22, 2003, while I was doing fieldwork on this very topic, a twenty-four-year-old youth did not resurface from jumping into a flooded mine quarry at Kit Hill, Callington.

My first exposure to jumping was also at a flooded mining site, on Carn Marth near Redruth, during the total eclipse of the sun on August 11, 1999. From 11:00 a.m. to 11:30 a.m., three men stripped down to their shorts and started jumping into the quarry. This eclipse provides a telling example of the confusion of appropriation by different groups within the Duchy, most specifically a confusion between commodified leisure pursuits and the cultivation of a local aura of mystery. The esoteric nature of the eclipse meant that an emphasis on creativity, rusticity, prehistory, and folklore took shape. By highlighting these themes, the promoters of and participants in the eclipse event were often unwittingly and sometimes consciously involved in a process of producing a regional aura of distinction – reinforcing the creation of social difference – elevating Cornwall to an otherworldly status. Jeff, an informant in his late thirties who was raised on the outskirts of Newquay and visits regularly from London, spoke for many when he said, "The eclipse is all about dying and being reborn. Unlike other artificial occasions, it's a natural form of emptying the old and bringing in the new. Time to start again, a once in a lifetime chance at self-purification."

The eclipse presented a chance to see something extraordinary and to be seen in extraordinary circumstances. Cornwall thus entered a quasi-liminal state for several days. If a pattern emerges from this disjointed discourse, it is perhaps that the eclipse helped reinforce the relationships between healing, death, society, and place. Indeed, the themes that conveyed themselves most coherently at the time orbited around how the moon's shadow over Cornwall for two minutes would provide the opportunity for a turning point at both personal and social levels. Considering this existential tension between death and rebirth, one could argue that these jumps were ceremonial – maybe even part of a pseudo-ritual. Partially at least, it seems that the jumps on this day were undertaken as a kind of symbolic social offering – or, as Stebbins (2007) would say, a form of leisure that is far from frivolous but is instead absolutely serious.

Of course, an alternative scenario could be proposed: that people jump off cliffs for little reason, simply because they are bored. In other words, that it is a meaningless act. The reply is itself simple – is not boredom a condition of existential angst that people strive to overcome? If people are lead to jump off cliffs because of their ennui, are they not engaging their social imaginations in some kind of ultimate search for a freedom from boredom? This brings up the idea of seeking "freedom" as in the term "free fall." Indeed, Bachelard's description of accession dreams and oneiric flight indicates the emancipatory potential of liberating oneself from earthly constraints: "A human being in his youth, in his taking off, in his fecundity, wants to rise up from the earth. The leap is a basic joy" (Bachelard [1943] 1988: 63).

Conversely, in *The Fall* Albert Camus (1956) points out how the action of falling is metaphorically entangled with many fundamental anxieties. For instance, the phenomenologist Mike Jackson (1996) illustrates how such idioms as "to loose one's footing," or "to be up in the air" figuratively convey insecurity and instability. We are thus led to question the kind of freedom the jumper is seeking. To a degree, I suspect that they are searching for the sensation of ultimate liberation of which such authors also speak. Hence, the goal of the cliff jumper can be seen to fit with the philosopher Bertrand Russell's maxim of living without certainty while avoiding the paralysis of hesitation (Russell in Slater 1997).

This is where Bachelard comes in again because it is not air that is dangerous to the jumper but the cliffs and the water. In another of Bachelard's influential works, *Water and Dreams: An Essay on the Imagination of Matter* ([1942] 1983), he provides a psychoanalytic/phenomenological framework for the understanding of water as a mediating substance between many things like life and death, surface and depth, the known and the unknown. The anthropologist Stuart McLean's (2003) recent work on bog mires in Ireland draws out some interesting ethnographic descriptions about the symbolism of water, some of which is reminiscent of Bachelard's observations. Indeed, in the present context, I am particularly compelled to elaborate on how they describe water as ubiquitous. If, as Bachelard suggests, the admixture of water and earth is one of the fundamental schemes of matter and materiality, is this not precisely because everything is in a fluid-like flux? Indeed, for Merleau-Ponty, the world and our bodies as perceived through the senses are also creative, shape shifting entities (Lakoff and Johnson 1999). We can thus perceive water through its metaphorical potential. Consequently, in the context that I have described in this article, it might be relevant to replace Merleau-Ponty's analogous connection that links the flesh of the body with "the flesh of the world," to an analogy in which our body as fluids connects with the fluids and the fluidity of the world.

Does this not point to a relationship with the healing properties of water? (Anderson 2002). Least we forget, of course, its possibilities for harm. Clearly these issues are important here. The fact that water surrounds most of Cornwall's borders alludes to a powerful visual metaphor about the role of crossing over water to reach the end of life. In this sense, many elderly migrants who take their retirement in Cornwall are often anticipating and preparing for death, crossing a threshold and embarking on a pilgrimage to the great beyond. Alternatively, what might be at work here is the fighting off of death.

Since the confrontation with death is an ultimate condition of existence, the relationship that cliff jumping has with death marks it out as a true existential act. In this sense, some people might be reminded of the act of jumping to intentionally end life. In both the case of jumping to live and jumping to die, the jumper is taking a risk of failure – the extreme sports enthusiast runs the risk of failing to execute the jump properly. Suicidal individuals also run the risk of failing to kill themselves. On a simple level, then, there could be two strands of jumps. In the first you have the young person who wants to feel life at its extreme, that is, jumping off a cliff for the pure rush and exhilaration. Some of the exhilaration comes once the jumper realizes that he or she has survived and they have proved to themselves that they are alive in the extreme. The antipode is the person for whom life itself has become too extreme. So much so that he or she can no longer stand to be alive; that is, no longer wants anything to do with the "extremity of life." Interestingly, reports of failed suicide attempts nevertheless suggest that a kind of euphoria comes over the person, perhaps given the knowledge or through the sensation that life is ending. Consequently, at the heart of each individual action there is a meeting point – existential extremity.

In both cases, a lot of planning can be involved. Yet spontaneity and a blurring of the distinction between accidents, jumping to live and jumping to die are frequently involved. Of particular relevance here is the engraving "The Suicide" by Thomas Rowlandson in the volume *The English Dance of Death* (1814–16). Brown (2001) describes this aquatint as an allegorical depiction. In it, Death sits passively and relishes the fact that his victims are doing his work for him – a man drowned in his attempt to save someone while his lover hurls herself into the turbulent sea to join him in death. Indeed, she chooses to kill herself but this choice is thrust upon her.

Jumping off high bridges or high structures in order to commit suicide or "show off" is an activity that has a rich history. Brown mentions the famous case of a daredevil in the nineteenth century who jumped off the Tower Bridge in London as a stunt and did not survive. More recently, the documentary *The Bridge* (2006) by Eric Steel also depicts the "popularity" of jumping as a means of attempting suicide. The filming at San Francisco's Golden Gate Bridge during 2004 reports an average of one person every fortnight jumping off the 220-feet-high suspension span with the intention of killing themselves. The Golden Gate remains the most frequent site for suicides in America, and thus ranks among the most prominent in the world, along with such places as the Aokigahara Forest at the base of Mount Fuji, Niagara Falls on the US/Canadian border, Paris's famous Eiffel Tower, the cliffs of Beachy Head in Sussex, and Brunel's Clifton Suspension Bridge in Bristol (the site of the first modern bungy jump on April 1, 1979 by the Dangerous Sports Club).

The public imagination was also caught by the well-known tragedy of "the falling man," whose image was depicted time and again. Hundreds of people jumped or were blown out of the Twin Towers on September 11, 2001. Of course, in these circumstances, we are no longer talking of suicide. Rather, it is a clear example of being pushed by circumstance. Some might even say that when faced with the inevitability of death, these jumpers were making a type of leap of faith, either for the unlikely chance of survival, or to catch one last breath, to live one last moment. This level of the absurd perhaps illustrates part of what Camus in *The Fall* ([1956] 1957) and Jean-Paul Sartre in *Being and Nothingness* (1956) are addressing in their own way. Given that at least one person was killed by being hit by such a falling victim during 9/11, we see an ironic paradox in the actual result of the jumps, not that I am suggesting the possibility of foresight in this case. Also, interestingly, we encounter some people's rejection of the possibility that their loved ones could have given up hope and actually "deliberately" leapt.

Conclusion: A Leap of the Imagination

In thinking about how Bachelard informs us on an anthropology of the imagination, I am much more in accord with his position on the dynamic imagination. With regard to the materiality of the elements, he shows a greater concern for the potential of an imagination that is embodied and embodying. Given the focus of this article on free-fall jumping into water from cliff faces, I am especially drawn to his evocations of verticality:

> it is in the *act itself*, lived as a unified whole, that dynamic imagination must be able to experience the double human destiny of depth and height. Dynamic imagination unites the two poles. It allows us to understand that something within us rises up when some action penetrates deeper – and that, conversely, something penetrates deeper when something else rises ... to stay closer to pure imagination – we are the strongest link between earth and air ... the earth and the air are, for a dynamized being, indissolubly linked. (1988: 108–9)

I would, of course, add, given the present context, that "the earth and air *and water* are, for the dynamized being, indissolubly linked." In terms of Merleau-Ponty's use of metaphorical embodiment, cliff jumping is thus a bodily metaphor for existence and identity. It provides a fleeting resolution of an existential struggle between locality and the global, freedom and constraint, modernity and nature (Lewis 2001). The body is rarely more unregulated than during these few moments of free-fall. So it is both the most natural and unnatural sensation since being truly free is unnatural.

As an event related to the creation and contention of identity and sociality, cliff jumping is clearly about performance. The dynamics governing cliff jumping are far more complex than that, however, since it is also about an intentional search for freedom through danger. There is a deliberate juxtaposition of a double reflexivity in the approach I have described. Hence, it is the study, writing, and narrating of the event that pushes cliff jumping beyond performance, to the level where it is a creative and imaginative act. An extreme practice of ontological and existential awareness.

No longer is jumping simply seen to be about performing identity or because it is just fun. Now jumping takes on relevance in relation to overcoming life's absurdities. It gives meaning and subverts the abstraction of the body. Additionally, given that it is dismissed by passed practitioners, jumping is a type of rite of passage, from youth to maturity, from insecurities to being settled. If, as Freud (1919) points out, the liberation of sexual repression is to die a little, then so too is the existential act of moving from adolescence to adulthood through the practice of cliff jumping. That is, jumping is also to die a little – to engage in a gradual process of sacrificing one's youth – one's adolescence.

In addition to the obvious relation to Merleau-Ponty's work on the phenomenology of the body, the practice of cliff jumping fits in nicely with the context of what Marcel Mauss calls "techniques of the body" ([1934] 1992) – corporal ways of being that become natural or normativized, but are also contingent, malleable, and allow for a creative physicality. Jumping is thus a material, symbolic, and imaginative act, a means of liberation and freedom, a search for the unknown. This brings forth the idea of appearance and aesthetics in jumping and falling. Here we can recall the television broadcast of "Jump London" on Channel 4 on September 9, 2003.

The processes of incorporating these techniques may be experienced as disciplining or punishing, as in Michel Foucault's (1977) description of the body: "they … mark it, train it, torture it, force it to carry out tasks, to perform ceremonies, to emit signs." Indeed, the modern body is one that recent scholarship often portrays as mechanized, surveyed, patrolled, and unintentionally subjected to risk thus never more regulated. Nevertheless, such techniques of the body can also be seen as therapeutic and emancipatory – vehicles for transporting the imagination. Hence, we need to ask whether corporeal regimentation is the only result of modernity, the only framework in which to consider risk taking? Or is there something else that is possible here? An alternative scenario that ethnography – perhaps inspired by multi-sited, postmodern, or phenomenological approaches – can pursue. A scenario in which the hazardous use of landscape when linked to positive encounters with danger, allows extreme acts to be interpreted beyond even the notions concerning performance, to a more far-reaching – perhaps "extremist" – position where some of them can be understood as existential acts of the social imagination (Laviolette forthcoming).

So, to come back to Kierkegaard, then, who has suggested that, when reason or poetics reach their logical extreme or creative end – when we are confronted with an intellectual impasse or an thwart of the imagination – a complete and all encompassing existential insecurity, we are forced into making some type of "leap of faith." That is, of devising an ontological means of continuing ([1843] 1983). The act of cliff jumping, as it exists in the realm of an embodied imagination, provides such a platform from which to take such creative leaps of faith.

Social scientists should thus be stretching the leaps of faith that we take in our interpretations, theorizing, and methodological approaches, especially with regard to the uncharted terrain of the role of the imagination in formulating our social and bodily identities. This means truly accepting that ethnographic practices are themselves inherently grounded in reflexivity, educated guesses, and calculated risks that allow us and our disciplines to survive, both in the perilous arenas of academia and in the hazardous world out there. In dealing with the interviewing, participation, and observation of such fleeting moments of euphoria that extreme activities provide, the researcher has necessarily reached a new methodological frontier. One of the most established ways we have of exploring this horizon is by the ethnographic practice of repeated participation, as well as the phenomenological process of detailed experiential description. These are indeed part of a more existentially based anthropological process of taking a fateful leap. In this case, such a leap is into the realm whereby landscape and nature, identity, the body, and the imagination come together through the cultural act of jumping off cliffs into water.

Acknowledgments

Earlier versions of this paper were presented on three occasions: at the Engaging Imagination conference on June 21, 2003 at DBS University College Dublin; at the Social Anthropology and Material Culture Seminar Series on December 3, 2003, University College London; and at the Sport and Anthropology Seminar, December 4, 2004, De Montfort University, Leicester. Thanks to the participants of these events for their suggestions. For their comments on earlier drafts, I am also grateful to Allen Abramson and Jean-Sébastien Marcoux.

References

Abramson, A. and P. Laviolette 2007. "Cliff-Jumping, World-Shifting and Value-Production: The Genesis and Cultural Transformation of a Dangerous New Game." *Suomen Antropologi: Journal of the Finnish Anthropological Society*, 32(2): 5–28.

Anderson, S.C. 2002. "Introduction: The pleasure of taking the waters." In Anderson, S.C. and B.H. Tabb. *Water, Leisure and Culture: European Historical Perspectives*. Oxford: Berg.

Bachelard, G. [1938] 1987. [La Psychanalyse du feu.] *The Psycho-analysis of Fire*. Translated by N. Frye. Dallas, TX: The Dallas Institute Publications.

Bachelard, G. [1942] 1983. [L'Eau et les rêves: essay sur l'imagination de la matière.] *Water and Dreams: An Essay on the Imagination of Matter*. Translated by E.R. Farrell. Dallas, TX: Pegasus Foundation.

Bachelard, G. [1943] 1988. [L'Air et les songes, essai sur l'imagination du movement.] *Air and dreams: An Essay on the Imagination of Movement*. Translated by E.R. Farrell. Dallas, TX: The Dallas Institute Publications.

Bachelard, G. [1947] 1988. [La Têrre et les reverie de la volonté, essay sur l'imagination de la matière.] *Earth and Reveries of Will: An Essay on the Imagination of Matter*. (K. Haltman). Dallas, TX: The Dallas Institute Publications.

Bell, C. and J. Lyall 2001. *The Accelerated Sublime: Landscape, Tourism and Identity*. Westport, CT: Praeger.

Brown, R. 2001. *The Art of Suicide*. London: Reaktion Books.

Busby, G. and P. Laviolette 2006. "Narratives in the Net: Fiction and Cornish Tourism." *Cornish Studies*. 14: 142–63.

Camus, A. [1956] 1957. *The Fall*. Translated by J. O'Brien. London: H. Hamilton.

Caplan, P. (ed.). 2000. *Risk Revisited*. London: Pluto Press.

Crang, P. 1997. "Regional Imaginations: An Afterword." In E. Westland (ed.), *Cornwall: The Cultural Construction of Place*. Penzance: Patten Press.

Dant, T. 1998. "Playing with Things: Objects And Subjects in Windsurfing." *Journal of Material Culture*. 3(1): 77–95.

Douglas, M. 1992. *Risk and Blame: Essays in Cultural Theory*. London: Routledge.

Ferrell, D. 2001. "Climbing Frozen Waterfalls." In D. Wimmer (ed.), *The Extreme Game: An Extreme Sports Anthology*. Short Hills, NJ: Burford Books.

Fernandez, J. and Huber, M.T. (eds.) 2001. *Irony in Action: Anthropology, Practice, and the Moral Imagination*. Chicago, IL: University of Chicago Press.

Fiske, J. 1989. *Reading the Popular*. London: Unwin Hyman.

Foucault, M. 1977. *Discipline and Punish: The Birth of the Prison*. Translated by A. Sheridan. New York: Vintage Books.

Freud, S. 1919. *Totem and Taboo*. London: Penguin.

Hunter, J. and M. Csikszentmihalyi 2000. "The Phenomenology of Body-Mind: The Contrasting Cases of Flow in Sports and Contemplation." *Anthropology of Consciousness*. 11(3/4): 5–25.

Husserl, E. 1931. *Ideas: General Itroduction to Pure Phenomenology*. Translated by W.R. Boyce-Gibson). London: George Allen & Unwin Ltd.

Ireland, M.J. 1989. "Tourism in Cornwall: An Anthropological Case Study." PhD dissertation. University of Swansea.

Jackson, M. (ed.). 1996. *Things as They Are: New Directions in Phenomenological Anthropology*. Bloomington, IN: Indiana University Press.

Jackson, M. 2005. *Existential Anthropology: Events, Exigencies and Effects*. Oxford: Berghahn Publishers.

Johnson, M. 1987. "Toward a Theory of Imagination. " In *The Body in the Mind: The Bodily Basis of Meaning, Imagination, and Reason*. Chicago, IL: Chicago University Press.

Karl F.R. and L. Hamalian (eds) [1963] 1973. Introduction. *The Existential Imagination*. London: Picador.

Kierkegaard, S. [1843] 1983. *Fear and Trembling/Repetition*. Edited and translated by H.V. Hong and E.H. Hong. Princeton, NJ: Princeton University Press.

Lakoff, G. and M. Johnson 1999. *Philosophy in the Flesh*. New York: Basic Books.

Laviolette, P. 2003. "Landscaping Death: Resting Places for Cornish Identity." *Journal of Material Culture*. 8(2): 215–40.

Laviolette, P. 2006a. "Ships of Relations: Navigating through Local Cornish Maritime Art." *International Journal of Heritage Studies*. 12(1): 69–92.

Laviolette, P. 2006b. "Green and Extreme: Free-Flowing through Seascape and Sewer." *Worldviews: Environment, Culture, Religion*. 10(2): 178–204.

Laviolette, P. 2007. Guest editorial: "Hazardous Sport?" *Anthropology Today*. 23(6): 1–2.

Laviolette, P. forthcoming. *Not a Hap-Hazardous Sport: Extreme Landscapes of Leisure*. Farnham: Ashgate.

Lewis, N. 2001. "The Climbing Body, Nature and the Experience of Modernity." In Macnaghten, P. and J. Urry (eds), *Bodies of Nature*. London: Sage Publications.

Lyng, S. 1990. Edgework: "A Socio Psychological Analysis of Voluntary Risk Taking." *American Journal of Sociology*. 95(4): 851–86.

Low, S. and D. Lawrence-Zuniga 2003. *The Anthropology of Space and Place: Locating Culture*. Oxford: Blackwell.

McLean, S. 2003. "Buried Landscapes of Childhood." In Strathern, A. and P.J. Stewart (eds). *Landscape, Memory and Identity*. London: Pluto Press.

Marcus, G. E. 1995. "Ethnography in/of the World System: The Emergence of Multi-Sited Ethnography." *Annual Review of Anthropology*. 24: 95–117.

Martin, R.B. 1980. *Tennyson, the Unquiet Heart: A Biography*. Oxford: Clarendon Press.

Mauss, M. [1934] 1992. "Techniques of the Body." In Crary J. and S. Kwinter (eds). *Incorporations*. New York: Zone Books.

Merleau-Ponty, M. 1962. *Phenomenology of Perception*. London: Routledge.

Slater, J. 1997. *Last Philosophical Testament, 1943–68 Volume 11*. London: Routledge.

Sartre, J-P. 1956. *Being and Nothingness: A Phenomenological Essay on Ontology*. (Trans. Barnes H. E.): Paris: Gallimard.

Schutz, A. 1970. *Alfred Schutz on Phenomenology and Social Relations*. Edited by H.R. Wagner. Chicago, IL: Chicago University Press.

Stebbins, R.A. 2007. *Serious Leisure: A Perspective for Our Time*. New Brunswick, NJ: Aldine/Transaction.

Steel, E. 2006. *The Bridge*. New York: Koch-Lorber Films.

Thornton, P. 1993. "Cornwall and Changes in the 'Tourist Gaze'." *Cornish Studies*. 1: 80–96.

Tilley, C. 1994. *A Phenomenology of Landscape: Places, Paths, Monuments*. Oxford: Berg Publishers.

Tuan, Y-F. 1974. *Topophilia: A Study of Environmental Perceptions, Attitudes, and Values*. Englewood Cliffs, NJ: Prentice Hall.

Tuan, Y-F. 1980. *Landscapes of Fear*. Oxford: Blackwell.

Senses & Society   VOLUME 4, ISSUE 3   REPRINTS AVAILABLE   PHOTOCOPYING   © BERG 2009
PP 323–344   DIRECTLY FROM THE   PERMITTED BY   PRINTED IN THE UK
PUBLISHERS   LICENSE ONLY

Embracing Sculptural Ceramics: A Lived Experience of Touch in Art

Bonnie Kemske

After ten years as a professional ceramist, Bonnie Kemske returned to education, gaining a PhD at the Royal College of Art for research into touch, tactility, and the body. Her "cast hugs" form part of the Assembling Bodies exhibition at the Museum of Archaeology and Anthropology, University of Cambridge running to November 2010. Examples of her artwork can be seen at www.bonniekemske.com. mail@bonniekemske.com

ABSTRACT   Sculptural ceramic objects created *by* and *for* the body were made within the context of art-based research, in which theoretical explorations and studio practice were integrally interwoven. Studio explorations developed from theoretical knowledge gained from human physiology, and from the development of an understanding of the "lived experience" as expressed by Maurice Merleau-Ponty, through the experiences of the artist in making, and comments from visitors at exhibitions. The artworks challenge the visual hegemony of the art gallery by more fully engaging the body's sense of touch through the embrace. The sculptures, which were made by "casting hugs," instinctively invite interaction, with soft curves that echo the human body, textures to visually entice

Senses & Society   DOI 10.2752/174589209X12464528171932

individuals to touch, and a pleasurable weight that slows down responses. In public exhibition the artworks are enthusiastically embraced and held, broadening and articulating a tactile aesthetic for sculpture, and shifting focus from the sculptural objects themselves to one's physical and emotional experience of those objects.

KEYWORDS: touch, tactile art, embrace, tactile aesthetic

I am sitting quietly in the small Japanese tearoom with my legs folded under me. The calm dimness rests my eyes and makes the muted natural amber colors of the room glow. The host sits in front of me. He pours hot water over the bright green tea he has placed in the ceramic tea-bowl. He rapidly whisks the tea to a froth, picks up the tea-bowl, turns it, and places it closer to me. I place the tea-bowl in front of myself, then exchange a bow with the host. I breathe. Then I carefully lift the tea-bowl into my left hand and feel the warmth of the tea spread through the ceramic bowl to fill my open palm. Molding my other hand around the side of the tea-bowl, I cradle the bowl that cradles the tea. I raise it slightly, bow almost imperceptibly, turn the tea-bowl two quarter turns, then raise its smooth rim to my lips.

Cradling the tea-bowl is not just a function in the Tea Ceremony; it serves as a synecdoche for the Tea Ceremony itself. It is deliberate and considered – imbued with consciousness, self-awareness, and shared action. It is the connection, tactile and spiritual, between you and the host, and the center of your own experience of this sensual art form.

Since this experience as a young Tea student in Japan, through ten years in the ceramics studio producing textured abstracted figurative work, and later as an artist-researcher, I have asked myself how I could capture the evanescent and self-reflective state achieved through the physical experience of Tea in sculptural ceramic objects. This paper tells of the part of this self-reflective journey undertaken as an artist-researcher, and of the experiences arising from it.

My work falls within the area of practice-based or art-based research, which comprises both theoretical and studio investigations, and which results in both critical text and artworks. There is ample support for this experiential model. In 1958 Michael Polanyi articulated the concept of "tacit knowing" as that which cannot be expressed or taught through language (Polanyi 1958). Since then, tacit knowledge has long been acknowledged and reflected upon within the craft and latterly the art world. Peter Dormer states, "Craft relies on tacit knowledge. Tacit knowledge is acquired through experience and it is the knowledge that enables you to do things as distinct from talking or writing about them" (Dormer 1997: 147). He expands this concept by considering the role of the craft practitioner within this "craft knowledge."

> Craft knowledge … has … a private aspect: craft knowledge resides in individual people. Such knowledge becomes a part of the self… In most complex crafts there is, for those expert in it, a form of dialogue going on between the practitioner, his expertise, and the goal that the practitioner is trying to make or find. (Dormer 1994: 18–19)

Art-based research had not yet developed during Dormer's time, but I believe that we can extend his understanding of the role of the practitioner to include that of the artist-researcher. Anna Fariello continues the discussion on tacit knowledge with this succinct summary: "While verbal language can provide clues to understanding and can stimulate reflection, it cannot replace knowing the work through experiential methods" (Fariello and Owen 2005: 155). Looking beyond craft theory, a recent book by sociologist Richard Sennett also supports the value of an experiential approach: "Good work … emphasizes the lessons of experience through a dialogue between tacit knowledge and explicit critique" (Sennett 2008: 51). In many ways art-based research well represents Sennett's vision of combining "tacit knowledge" as practice, and "explicit critique" as theory. The artwork created as part of this research could not have developed without the fundamental interweaving of practice and theory.

Touch and Tactility

For many years I had been producing tactile textured ceramic forms as a studio artist. As an artist-researcher I chose to begin the research into tactility, again in a studio setting. I first considered how I might encourage individuals to engage physically with artworks through the qualities of the artwork itself. If I offered them textures that were visually alluring, would they be tempted to touch to verify the quality of the surface? I devised a project to establish which clays and firing temperatures would be most tactilely pleasing. I created almost one hundred identically textured tiles in various clays and fired them to different temperatures. However, it became clear very early on that there was no universal tactile aesthetic to be found. The tiles were rated differently by myself and others, and rated differently again in a second rating. Research by Charles Spence confirms the changing nature of tactile perception. Spence showed that a texture was commonly rated as rougher if the subject being tested heard the sound of sandpaper being scraped while touching the texture (Spence 2004). Our senses are multidimensional and interdependent.

The Role of Touch

What is touch? I needed to understand the role of touch in our lives theoretically, and to reflect on it personally. This led me to understand touch as our most direct, least intellectualized, sense. It is the grounding sense, the sense of tangibility that places us in the world. As the full proverb states, "Seeing is believing, but feeling is the truth" (attributed to British clergyman Thomas Fuller, 1608–61). Yet it seems to me that within our Western culture a hegemony of vision erodes our tactile sensitivities.

In Tiffany Field's book *Touch* she stated that within our Western culture many of us are touch deprived, and she refers to this as "touch hunger" (Field 2001: 1–17). A quick survey of popular culture illustrates how we search for new ways to incorporate touch in our lives. There are massage chairs, belts, and pillows. Health spas provide access to saunas and jacuzzis. Showers have settings to stimulate the skin. And there are more and more types of massage on offer – shiatsu, Swedish, Reiki, and Rolfing among others. All these things can be seen as ways of increasing personal touch stimulation in our tactile hungry society.

How much touch we need, how we perceive touch, whether we find it pleasant or distasteful, and how we react to it, vary dramatically from person to person. It is influenced by factors such as our genetic make-up, experiences as a fetus, baby, child, and adult, our gender, the attitudes and mores of our society, our personal circumstances, and our emotional and physical state at any one time. So although touch is a universal experience, it is also an utterly intimate and individual one.

Touch in Art

In the world of fine art in the twentieth century, partly as a backlash against movements such as Formalism (from Russian Formalism through to Abstract Expressionism), with its preoccupation with the visual aspects of color, form, line, and composition, artists such as those working within the Arte Povera movement led the way to more fully engaging our senses through their use of non-traditional materials, often mundane materials with which we interact daily (Lumley 2004). This type of work began to challenge the no-touching policies within museums and galleries, and in the past few years curators and gallery owners have been grappling with practical as well as conceptual issues surrounding touching artwork (see Heritage Studies Research Group 2004). Indeed, galleries and museums have recently mounted exhibitions aimed at engaging touch. Three examples in London alone can be given. The Victoria and Albert Museum's exhibition entitled *Touch Me: Design and Sensation* (V&A 2005) specifically set out to challenge the anti-touch status quo, and included work by international applied artists. Within this exhibition there were many design items with which visitors could interact, the emphasis seeming to be more on interaction itself than on any tactile experience of the displays. The University for the Creative Arts hosted an exhibition entitled *"HAPTIC: Awakening the Senses"* (UCA 2008), which tried to engage the visitor's sense of touch by providing small touchable samples of the materials used in the artworks. However, this still forced the visitor to rely on touch memory to have a sense of touching the artwork. For *Jerwood Contemporary Makers* (Jerwood 2008), seven artists from differing craft disciplines were asked to produce work on the theme of touch on the physical, imagined, and metaphorical levels. Of the work of the seven artists, visitors were allowed to actually touch only one artwork, Clare Twomey's *Witness*, a wall covered with porcelain dust onto which visitors were welcomed to leave their mark. In the remainder of the exhibition we were asked to accept what our eyes told us, to experience the tactile qualities of the works secondhand, through vision and words. Even though the exhibition was themed "touch," ironically, it left a sense of touch deprivation, the experience remaining anticipative and unconsummated (Kemske 2008: 26). These exhibitions demonstrate that curators did not or chose not to consider the multiple aspects of touch, leaning heavily on single understandings – respectively, interaction, touch as visual verification, and touch as imagined or metaphorical.

The Materiality of Clay

It was particularly surprising to find such extreme restrictions on actual touching in the Jerwood exhibition because, through function and utility, crafts or applied arts have historically been the touchable arts. This long history of handling ceramics objects was part of the basis of my decision to situate this research within the field of sculptural ceramics. I feel the familiarity of the material helps us to overcome our reservations about touching artwork. In addition, fired clay has physical properties that are particularly suitable for tactile exploration. It is hard, yet can feel responsive to our touch, partly because it can absorb our body heat. It is a material that enticingly embraces contrast. It can be rough or smooth or both simultaneously. Its heaviness can be perceived as comforting. In addition, it never loses the echo of its making; it is a frozen moment that embodies the act of its creation, a permanent link between maker and the person holding the artwork. I believe that as humans we have an innate and intimate familiarity with and sensitivity to fired clay.

Touch and the Body

I decided to find out more about the mechanics of touch, or how the body touches, which led to a working understanding of the body's physiology and neurophysiology. It was the Two-Point Discrimination Threshold Test that led me to fully understand and appreciate that touch is not a single sense and that our experience of touch is very different across different parts of our bodies. This test is used clinically to indicate neurological damage. It also identifies normal differences in sensation. In the test the individual has his or her eyes shut or covered. A two-pointed caliper-like instrument is pressed against the skin on different parts of the body, both points being applied simultaneously. The person indicates whether or not he or she perceives the contact as two distinct points or as a single point. The distance between the two points is made larger and smaller over a series of touchings until a "threshold" is determined, that is, the widest measurement at which the person still perceives two points to be one.

The differences across the body can be extreme. For instance, the skin of the fingertip and lip is very sensitive, whereas the thigh, forearm, and back is not (Sinclair 1981: 180). Acknowledging the need to evaluate the tactile sensations personally, I had my own two-point discrimination thresholds tested. Figure 1 demonstrates the extreme variations. On my fingertip I perceived any two points closer together than 3 millimeters to be one point, whereas on my thigh it was 42 millimeters. Indeed, my own two-point discrimination thresholds are in fact rather more acute than average. This may be one of the reasons I am drawn to the field of touch, or perhaps I have become sensitized through the heightened awareness resulting from my work.

Using the results of this test I produced small hand-held textured ceramic forms to be run across the body, creating varying sensations. One particularly successful piece was made to be run down the inside of the arm, evoking a variety of sensations as it traveled across the different sensitivities of the upper and lower arm, wrist, palm, and fingers. If it were not for the continuity of the touch, the same object would feel like many different objects as it travels over the skin.

I found that individuals willingly engaged with these pieces when invited to do so. However, their interactions with them were rapid, both in the speed of their actions and in the length of time they spent in exploration. I felt this discouraged a positive reflective experience, such as the one I had had in Japanese Tea Ceremony, and thought larger works might both increase the length of time people took with each piece and slow down their responses.

Looking again at the physiology of touch led to understanding touch not as singular, but as a manifold experience. Distinct receptors have the abilities to perceive and discriminate pressure, texture, vibration, hot, cold, a light touch (Olausson, Lamarre, Backlund et al., 2002: 900–4), and pain, which includes itch and tickle, and the densities and distribution of these receptors vary across the body. I decided to try to incorporate the multiple senses of touch into the work.

To determine how I might do this, I revisited earlier research I had done into how different cultures interact tactilely with ceramics. I recalled a conversation with Nigel Barley, anthropologist and author, at the British Museum (Barley 1994), about women potters in Africa who make pots to fit their bodies to facilitate carrying. I intended

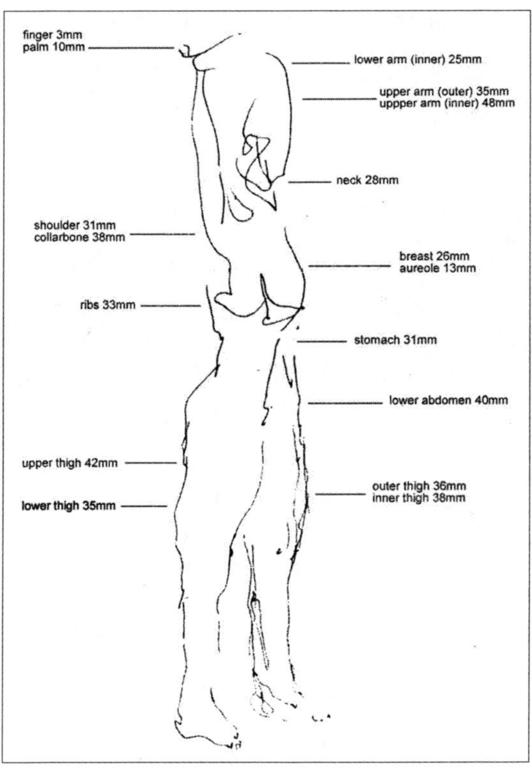

Figure 1
The artist's two-point discrimination thresholds: the widest point at which two points applied to the skin simultaneously are perceived as a single point (in millimeters).

my work to be sculptural, not functional, but I thought that creating artworks that fit the body might be one way to try to more fully engage our sense of touch.

Touching Beyond the Hand

First, I had a plaster cast made of my own body. I built sculptures upon the cast that would then fit against my body. I then textured the surfaces of the forms, using coarse textures where the sculptures rested against the body and fine textures for areas that the hands would have access to. The resultant objects fit snugly against different parts of my body. However, during a three-month period of working in Japan, I had no body cast, so I built the objects directly on my own body, that is, I shaped plastic clay against my bare skin, using my body as a mold. This experience was challenging, but also physically engaging, and led me to reflect about my relationship to the pieces I was creating. Here are extracts from journal notes made during the making experience:

- The clay is cool but warms quickly.
- Feels snug, contained, comfortable – caressed?
- There's a strong sense of immediacy and intimacy.
- A single perspective – an inner perspective of tactile experience.
- Until I lift it away from my body it exists solely as part of me.

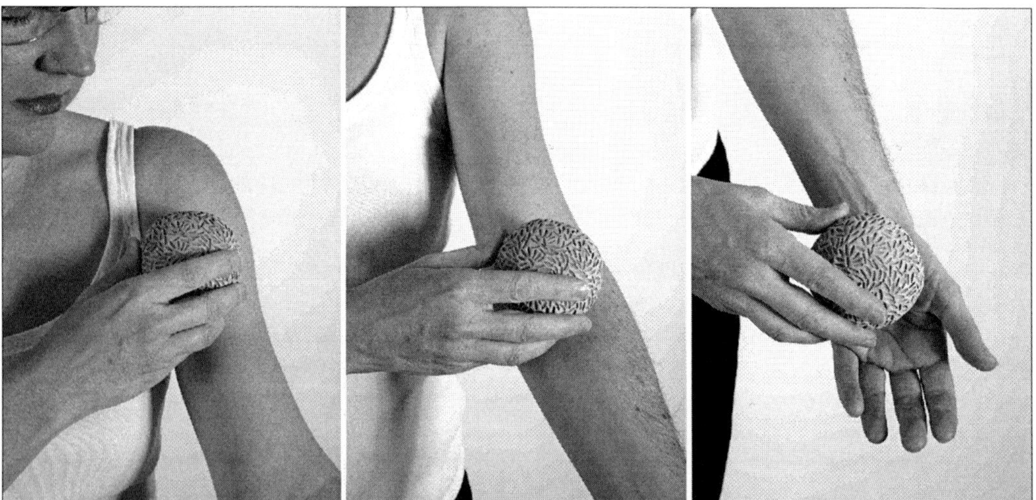

Figure 2
Running a textured artwork down the inside of the arm to create differing sensations.

■ This piece is an object to me (the subject), but why doesn't it feel like that?

Being in Japan I looked to Japanese philosophy to understand my experience. It was the work of Japanese philosopher Nishida Kitarō that made me begin to think of the making process as experience, rather than just a way to reach the end-point. Nishida says, "To experience means to know events precisely as they are. It means to cast away completely one's attitude of discriminative reflection, and to know in accordance with the events" (Nishida cited in Encyclopædia Brittanica 2007). This is what he calls "pure experience," a "direct" experience prior to the separation of subject and object (Nishida 1990: 48), a moment of pre-intellectualization.

> In pure experience, our thinking, feeling, and willing are still undivided; there is a single activity, with no opposition between subject and object. Such opposition arises from the demands of thinking, so it is not a fact of direct experience. In direct experience there is only an independent, self-sufficient event, with neither a subject that sees nor an object that is seen. (Nishida 1990: 48)

The deeper engagement of my body within the experience of making served as a good example to me of this kind of "direct experience." I created three pieces in this way and exhibited them in a public art gallery in Kyoto. Finding a way to display the sculptures to encourage touching forced me to consider the role of the gallery and setting.

Touch in the Gallery

No matter what has gone into the creation of the specific artwork, the pieces can never be considered outside their context, and one's

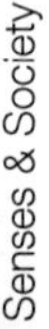

first encounter with an artwork is most often within a gallery setting. When entering a museum or gallery the sign one is most likely to see reads: Do Not Touch. The sign fortifies the social taboo against touching artwork, but it also serves as a signal to us that there *is* something there to touch, some encounter to be experienced beyond visual engagement. The sign both prohibits us from touching and challenges us to reach out and run a finger over the surface of the art object.

Curators and exhibition designers often reinforce the no-touch policy through the creation of gallery spaces that are dramatic and memorable by using minimal display, specifically designed lighting, and strong focal points. These design qualities, and the reverential hush that accompanies them, often evoke a sense of the church or temple, especially when the artwork is displayed on a plinth, which may evoke images of the altar.

What does this no-touch policy "do" for the artwork? Where there are large numbers of exhibition visitors there can be protective benefits for delicate or valuable artworks; the social taboo can help prevent breakage, soiling, and can deter theft. The placing of the artwork on a plinth also changes its signification; it informs us that the piece has a considerable monetary and/or cultural value, and it also raises the perceived status of the artist. In addition, not touching precludes individuals from having to know how to physically engage with an artwork, keeping them from the social embarrassment of mishandling the work. It also reinforces elitism within the art world by declaring that "we" in the art world (makers, curators, collectors) may handle the artwork, whereas "they" (the public) may not.

In the Kyoto exhibition people did interact with the artworks, but not as I expected. I thought they would fit the works to their bodies in the same positions in which I had made them, but people interacted with them in numerous and creative ways, engaging with them very personally and intimately.

Into the Lived Experience

Looking to expand my understanding of the intimacy and immediacy of the making, the sense of the work being part of me as I formed it, and the blur I felt between me as subject and the artwork as object, I looked to the French phenomenologist Maurice Merleau-Ponty to try to understand conceptually what was happening in this experience. I carried his concepts of an inseparable mind and body, the "incarnated mind," and the "double belongingness" of simultaneously touching and being touched with me into the next stage of making and wrote and reflected on it during that time.

It was clear that I needed to continue to make work using my body, but now I wanted to try to create forms that had no conscious design element, forms that were derived solely from my body's own involvement. I was also concerned that in the artworks I had created thus far, the visual aspects were still dominant. In looking for a way to

Figure 3
Visitors interacting with
artwork at an exhibition in
Kyoto, Japan.

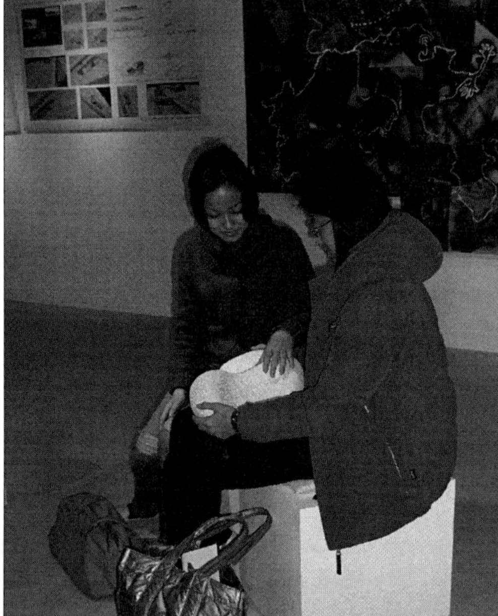

fully engage the body, I came to "cast hugs," that is, I sat or lay in the studio embracing a large plaster-filled latex balloon until it set.

In this way I overrode my training in the visual aesthetic, using instead only my tactile senses. The works were created through three determinants alone: my body, the state of the plaster, and the sizes of the balloons. After casting a series of "hugs," when deciding which hugs to further develop into artworks, I first chose those casts that were pleasurable to touch and hold. Secondly, I looked for shapes that might visually entice us to physically engage with the artwork through touching, lifting, handling, and caressing.

I then made molds of the cast hugs and used them to reproduce the shapes in clay, texturing the finished forms, firing, then applying a surface of terra sigillata, which is a fine slip or liquid clay, before a final low firing.

Touch and the Embrace

Touch is the first sense to appear in the developing fetus and the last sense to leave (Montagu 1986: 3). As soon as the fetus is large enough, the embrace of the womb is one of the first experiences of touch it has. After birth, infants who are not touched and embraced suffer many disturbing and debilitating conditions, including stunted growth and aggressive behavior (Field 2001: 59–74). Adults as well as children need significant touch experiences in their lives (Field 2001: 91–115) and regular hugging can help people have healthier hearts, especially women (Light, Grewen, and Amico 2005: 5–21).

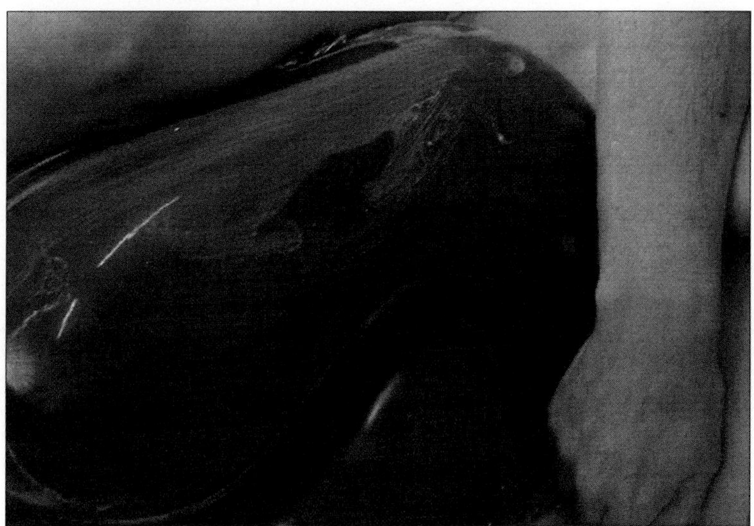

Figure 4
Close-up image of the
process of casting hugs.

We can embrace and be embraced throughout our lives, and the embrace is clearly seen as a positive experience. The Free Hugs Movement video (www.freehugscampaign.org), which shows a man on the street and in shopping malls giving hugs, still circulates on the internet, and is enacted from time to time around the world. Cuddle Parties have been reported in the media (Lusher 2006; see also www.cuddleparty.com). These hugging parties, which originated in New York, are now being enacted in several countries. A cross-over with health, well-being, and religious issues can be seen in the phenomenon that is Mata Amritanandamayi – Amma. The laying-on of hands is a common religious activity, especially within some Christian sects; what distinguishes Amma from other spiritual healers is her specific use of the embrace.

> They came by the thousands, from the city and from all over the country, just looking for a hug. But Mata Amritanandamayi – known to her devotees as Amma – is no ordinary hugger. The 50-year-old woman from India, who wears a white sari and a diamond-studded nose ring, is nicknamed the Hugging Saint for the embraces that have earned her a worldwide following. By early yesterday morning, more than 2,000 people had packed the hall at the Manhattan Center on W. 34th St., eager for a moment in the arms of the spiritual guru. (Lebovich cited in Classen 2005: 106)

Extensive field research and the use of methods such as focus groups have given major advertisers an edge on knowing what the public wants. A notable campaign advertising Orange mobile telephones used scenes of young people hugging. An international company as large as Orange using the hug as a marketing image, is a clear indication that hugging is of significant relevance to their young adult target audience.

Age, however, does not seem to deter the need for the embrace. Rose Hacker, a 101-year-old newspaper columnist, wrote,

> Being hugged is the fulfillment of the dream. My parents never touched us – we had a peck on the cheek at most. When my father died, however, he held out his arms from the bed and cried "Rosie darling." That was the only time he ever hugged me, and I remember thinking: "I've been wanting this all my life." (Hacker 2007: 10–11)

The Art of the Experience

Building on my making experience and understanding the embrace led me to realize that the "art" of the artwork I was producing was not manifest in the material object itself, but rather in the individual's experience of the object. As Merleau-Ponty said, "What is given is not the thing on its own, but the experience of the thing." (Merleau-Ponty 1962: 379) I do not consider the works to be complete until they are held against the body.

At this point it was clear to me that I needed to acknowledge, develop, and chronicle the significance of the making experience. To more fully integrate and reflect on the concepts I was grappling with and the experience of making, I wrote of the experience, intertwining the physicality of the experience with reflections on Merleau-Ponty's writings.

The use of my own body in the making of these artworks had become important, but I did not know how this related to other people's responses to the finished work. My desire was not to have others simply replicate the experience of making. Many of us have felt the thrill of fitting our fingers into the making marks left by the potter of an ancient vessel, but I felt strongly that this "replication" was not what I sought. Touch is a universal experience, but ultimately, it is also personal and individual, and I wanted each encounter with an artwork to evoke an individual's response drawn from his or her own personal history, not to serve as a personal communication from me as maker to the individual as receiver.

So how did an individual's experience of the work compare and relate to my experience of making? In exhibition I had discovered that, although people did not physically fit the artworks to their own bodies as I had in making, did not in fact "replicate" the making, I could deduce from the written and spoken comments I collected from visitors during exhibitions, that we did, in fact, share many of the same emotional and physical experiences. Correlating those comments to the emergent writing style I had developed as a way to bring together my experience of making with my understanding of Merleau-Ponty, I will explore seven themes that arose.

The Thoughtful Body

> *Sitting on the floor, holding a plaster-filled latex balloon against my bare skin until it sets… My ankle is pinned beneath the shifting mass that rests on top of it, engulfed by the weight of the soft plaster as it oozes around and over the hardness of bone. I center it to my torso, holding its confined fluidity in place with my legs and arms.*
>
> "It is through my body that I go to the world," wrote Merleau-Ponty. This could not be more evident than now, as I press my body around this moving, oozing weight. I understand my perception of this mass in terms of Merleau-Ponty's "lived experience," an experience of and through the body. But Merleau-Ponty's body is not simply a collection of physiological assets; it is inseparable from the mind, just as the mind cannot be considered independently of the body. "The perceiving mind is an incarnated mind" (Merleau-Ponty 2004: 34). Thought and corporeality together are the whole. All I perceive/feel/think is grounded in this, my conscious body, the thoughtful body. It is "the general instrument of my 'comprehension'" (Merleau-Ponty 1962: 273).

There were differing ways that Merleau-Ponty's "lived experience" and "incarnated mind" were expressed by visitors. Some individuals directly linked body and mind in statements such as "It's fascinating – and relaxing… It helps you think because it gives you something to touch and handle" or "The continuous texture is safe and let's you explore it to find new ways – an analogy for new patterns in life." Also, I believe that statements that indicate a sense of self in relation to the physical experience can express these Merleau-Ponty concepts as well. Visitors used the words "intimate," "personal," "sensual," "calming," and "quiet," words that serve as expressions of self-awareness of states of being that transcend the separation of mind and body as they express both simultaneously. Another good example can be seen in the comment of one man: "I feel I should be weeping, having a breakdown, like it's drawing it out of me."

Overlapping or Encroachment

> *I move my ankle and feel the unstable liquid roll slightly back and forth within its own weight. Squeezing my legs together, my right thigh presses into the heavy liquid, which is surprisingly resistant.*

> "There is overlapping or encroachment, so that we must say that the things pass into us as well as we into the things" (Merleau-Ponty 1968: 123). I feel the heavy liquid move against my thigh and its resistance to the pressure I impose on it. The liquid mass is distorting, as much as molding to my body, which dents, dimples, and alters under the form's weight. For me, this experience goes beyond Merleau-Ponty's description of an overlapping or encroachment. At this moment I and the embraced form exist only in relation to each other. We connect in an intimate and ever-shifting state of interaction and share influence on each other and presence in the world.

The comment "You transform something hard and unyielding into something soft, smooth, inviting and irresistible" expresses a state of interaction between body and artwork that is reflective of Merleau-Ponty's "encroachment," as does "As soon as I fit it to my body and found a place where it was comfortable, it didn't feel cold or hard anymore." Transformation expresses the influence that occurs between body and the object being held; each transforms the other. Engagement also signifies a taking in, an encroachment, in comments such as "It drew me to it," "It makes you want to lean into it," and "As sculptural objects these are beautiful, they are also visually very inviting. You want to touch and hold them." Finally, many people indicated that when embracing the artworks they developed a sense that the objects had become part of themselves. "Pressing the curvaceous shape into my body felt as if I was hugging an extension of myself" and "It's so soothing – it sort of melts into your body" are good examples of this.

The Shared Boundary

> *The squeeze of my legs moves the skin of my inner thigh across the smooth texture of the mass, an intimate contact that triggers my awareness of its slippery surface. My now-slippery thigh slides over its surface.*
>
> Now which is slippery? The form or my inner thigh? And where is the line between me and it? A viscous blur. 'It is as though our vision were formed in the heart of the visible, or as though there were between it and us an intimacy as close as between the sea and the strand. And yet it is not possible that we blend into it, nor that it passes into us' (Merleau-Ponty 1968: 130–1).

Merleau-Ponty's words refer to vision but I can extrapolate them to include touch. The viscous blur is the connection between me and the mass I perceive, an intimate and integral interface that joins me and it. Yet it is more than merely a shared boundary, a dividing membrane.

A concept closely related to that of encroachment is the blurred or shared boundary between subject (me as maker or an individual as embracer) and object (the sculptural artworks). Some visitor comments addressed this directly, as in "It's requited – it touches you – you and the work absorb each other" and "At first it feels cold, but very quickly you can feel it becoming warm. And as you move your hands over it, you can feel where you've been holding it. So you have a sense of how you are changing it as much as it is affecting you. It's responsive." Others express it in terms of their own bodies: "I am astonished by the way these rock-like works fit so lovingly around all the curves, the places of my body. They are cool to the touch, and appeal to the sensual, maternal aspects of my being. They are marvelously feminine, voluptuous and strangely comforting" and "I like the way the hardness makes me move around and fit my body to it, rather than the other way around. It makes me aware of muscles and my body that I'm not normally aware of."

The "and" between Subject and Object

> *Shifting forward I press my left forearm into the top of the amorphous mass. It makes only a subtle impression. So I lock my right hand onto my left wrist and bear down again. My arm sinks into the firmness a little more.*
>
> My arm presses in, and in doing so, becomes both sensor and agent, "the body as sensible and the body as sentient" (Merleau-Ponty 1968: 136). It both feels and acts. "Our body is a being of two leaves, from one side a thing among things and otherwise what sees them and touches them; … it unites these two properties within itself, and its double belongingness to the order of the 'object' and to the order of the 'subject' reveals to us quite unexpected relations between the two orders" (Merleau-Ponty 1968: 137). It is in these dual roles, within this double belongingness, that Merleau-Ponty explores the "and" between sensible and sentient, subject and object, passive and active – two manifestations of the same body – one experience. As I try to impress my body into the changing shape, I am aware of my double belongingness. I feel the mass's physical and independent presence, but I also feel my influence on its very existence.

The "and" between subject and object is manifest in many forms. First, there is the direct influence of the body on the object and the object on the body in comments like "It's cooling my chest, but warming where my hands are" and "Because it is ceramic I expected it to be hard and cold. And it was, as long as I was handling it. But as soon as I fit it to my body and found a place where it was comfortable, it didn't feel cold or hard anymore." Then there are comments that differentiate between self and object at the same time as expressing another kind of inseparable "double belongingness." This can be seen in the comment "It's about me but at the same time it's about this object." Finally, I believe that some of the more ambiguous comments that express a sense of contradiction may also reflect the "and." This can be seen in "Soft, hard, squashy, resilient – need to touch them!" "Oddly comfortable – strangely comforting," "Intuitively you think it won't feel very nice because it's hard and heavy, but it feels good, it's soothing," and "Isn't it amazing that something so hard can feel so soft?"

Chiasm

> *Curling over its bulk I add the weight of my upper body to the squeeze. My breasts sink down. I feel the discomfort of their flattened distortion, yet they make only shallow valleys in the shifting mass.*
>
> My body is both touching and being touched by the mass I enfold. Awareness shifts from one to the other – toucher to touched, touched to toucher – with little control on my part. This shift is Merleau-Ponty's chiasm, the "and." It is "the motion of perpetual dehiscence, in which perception is understood as a being in momentum" (Vasseleu 1998: 30). Enclosing this mass within the confines of my arms, legs, and torso leads me to understand that this dehiscence, which is defined as both a gaping and a bursting forth, can be seen as experience itself, a cusp of continuous and never-completed change. "The idea of *chiasm* [is] that … every relation with being is *simultaneously* a taking and a being taken, the hold is held, it is *inscribed* and inscribed in the same being that it takes hold of" (Merleau-Ponty 1968: 266). The chiasm isn't a mechanism, a switch to be thrown that will change one perspective to another. It is the experience of perception, "the organic relationship between subject and world, the active transcendence of consciousness" (Merleau-Ponty 1962: 176).

One visitor on leaving the exhibition area remarked, "I feel like I've still got it against me." Another said, "It's almost like your mother. It makes me feel comfortable. I've got, like, a bond with it now. When I'm not hugging it, it feels wrong." I think these two comments express Merleau-Ponty's concept of simultaneous touching and being touched in that the absence of the object identifies the "being touched" that had been experienced while caressing the artwork. Then there is the sense of the incomplete or never-ending. This can be seen in comments where the action is seen as indefinite or ongoing, such as "First you slide your hand all over, then you begin to find the dimples. I just want to explore them. I go back to them again and again." Another comment also reflects touch as process, rather than as static: "It's calming and quiet. The texture makes you go into the piece – want to feel the wabi-sabi imperfections. The smoothness feels too hard – you search for the imperfections. The texture makes you explore it."

Communication/Communion/Community

I ease back slightly and immediately feel the rounded shape reform. I press again and this time the emerging form nudges downward. The bulge nudges against my pubic bone.

This sensual nudge evokes unstructured yet familiar sensations, not exactly memories, but feelings I associate with warmth, comfort, and an accompanying suggestion of arousal. "Every perception is a communication or a communion, the taking up or completion by us of some extraneous intention, or on the other hand, the complete expression outside ourselves of our perceptual powers and a coition, so to speak, of our body with things" (Merleau-Ponty 1962: 373).

I focus on maintaining this hug, my thighs squeezed together, my body curled over, and my arms and breasts forcefully pressing down into the thickening form of the hug.

Is this Merleau-Ponty's communication/communion? "I am able to touch effectively only if the phenomenon finds an echo within me, if it accords with a certain nature of my consciousness, and if the organ which goes out to meet it is synchronized with it" (Merleau-Ponty 1962: 369). There is an unspoken experience of synchronization, of communion, of finding the echo inside of me. I sit with this hug held within the circle of my body and feel the many echoes of experience – echoes of safety, of sexual tension, of great joy, of maternal longing, of motherly love. At this transient, ever-incomplete moment the thickening form and my perception of it coalesce with/within me, my own perception part of the conversation. Yet this is a softly-defined completion, a fullness of uncertainty.

The heavy form my body cradles is quickening and becomes warm against my skin. Ironically, it quickens into solidity. I shift slightly and the stiffening weight no longer follows me. It no longer oozes around me and hugs me; its movement is stilled. I must now press myself around it to maintain the embrace. I become the one who moves.

Another layer of the chiasm, being on the edge of one thing, but continuously being and becoming its opposite, being and becoming neither, the incompleteness. This incompleteness has a depth that avows that there is no purely physical sensation or purely mental reflection. Each sensation/thought is embedded in a resonance within me that creates the perception, encompassing all that sensation is: spiritual, emotional, mental, physical…

This "resonance" can be specific in association as in the comments: "It makes me feel sleepy. Maybe that's because I need something heavy on me to fall asleep. The weight feels safe and reassuring. It feels significant. Also, the texture is important. It feels right. Calming. It wouldn't work if they were soft. The hardness feels strong, safe"; "It reminds me of large stones in my village in Iran where women in labor press their bodies against the stone to take away the pain. Also, we have stones that we believe take our emotional pain away. We say then that the stone is crying"; and "The curves of the objects made me think of my family when I touched them, and gave me tears. A very warm feeling." In these instances the experience of caressing the artwork has evoked particular memories or associations that are separate from the artwork. However, although the resonance within an individual's history is still apparent, some visitor comments also demonstrate that a new association can be created. This can be seen in the following examples: "It makes me feel slightly more important because now I have a purpose, I am looking after something important"; "It wants to be held – it doesn't want to be put back in its box"; "The big smooth one feels like you have to look after it. The others feel like they're looking after you"; and "I feel that the textured ones reject me."

These last comments also point to an interesting anthropomorphizing of the artworks that was also evident in other comments from visitors.

Towards an understanding

> *The gliding of my hand across the surface, the squeeze of my thighs to hold it in place, the press of my breasts and torso against the now well-defined form…*
>
> Perception is not passive; it is the "lived experience," a direct participation between me and the world.

Completing the circle we arrive back at the "lived experience." Comments like "Without thinking, I stroke it against my cheek. The smooth and meandering surfaces and their weight are just right"; "It fits. I just want to wrap my arms around it"; and "When you get it in the right place, it works. It rests on you, feels comfortable" give a sense of the interaction with the artwork as one that engages mind and body only as an integral experience, where the physical sensations evoke emotional feelings that in turn reinforce the corporal.

The Embrace as a Shared Experience

Visitors' comments also point to aspects of the experience that I did not envision or anticipate. Individuals and family members used the artwork to express and perhaps to strengthen bonds, such as a father who embraced a child who embraced a sculpture, or a mother who embraced her daughter, and an adult daughter who embraced her mother. The embracing of the artwork became a shared experience, as one visitor expressed it:

> The hug is about a closeness, of sharing an emotional charge. I feel like I am getting the charge from all the people who have hugged this before me. It's important that it's been hugged before – that it's a shared hug. The hug gives you emotional energy.

Another visitor put it this way:

> Snuggling up next to an object that "fits" with your body – quite intimate yet strange, as you are not the only person who "fits" with that object … it's like sharing the same intimate moment – that is experienced by many others but at different times in different places – people with different associations, experiences and backgrounds.

Finally, many visitors addressed the hug directly, giving support to the project and the making of sculptural ceramic objects to be embraced. Three examples include "So comforting! Hugs are the most special thing in my life!" "I can see that they would fit anyone

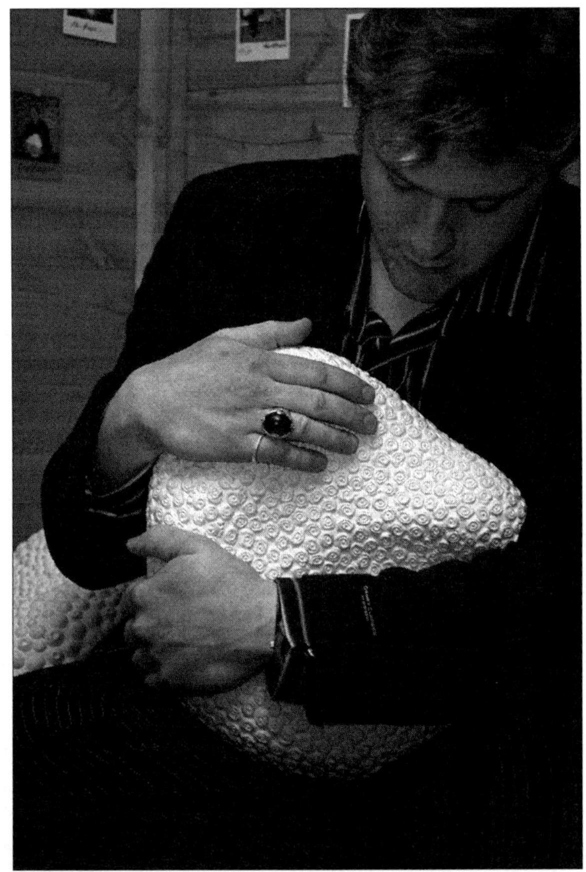

– after all, hugs fit everyone," and "The hardness of the ceramic is interesting – like a hug. A hug is soft but strong and firm too."

The experience of casting hugs led me to understand the embrace as a positive and transforming "lived experience." Visitor comments suggest that they too experienced much the same in their physical interaction with the artworks. I believe that for both maker and embracer the ever-flowing merging and shifting between touching and being touched, and the blurring of the boundary between the body and the object it holds, results in a slide of awareness from the "object" to the "experience of the object." The mind and body, integrally embedded in each other, experience a bodily pleasure that is inseparable from an emotional or intellectual pleasure.

An On-Going Ending

The sculptural artworks I have created aim to engage the body's sense of touch through corporal interaction. Visitors' comments showed that physical encounters with the sculptures could evoke sensual responses that were both emotional and physical. This was achieved through exploiting a sense of the familiar at the same time as offering tactile and visual enticement with new shapes and textures. The moment of fitting the sculpture to the body within the embrace brought forth a consonance of heightened physical and emotional self-awareness, an engagement of "the thoughtful body."

A gallery setting. A woman sits with the sculptural ceramic object on her lap. She settles it comfortably across her thighs, then explores its surface. She lifts the piece and holds it against her torso. Her arms cradle it.

References

Barley, Nigel. 1994. *Smashing Pots: Works of Clay from Africa*. Washington, DC: Smithsonian Institution Press.

Classen, Constance (ed.). 2005. *The Book of Touch*. Oxford: Berg.

Dormer, Peter. 1994. *The Art of the Maker*. London: Thames and Hudson.

Dormer, Peter. 1997. "Craft and the Turing Test for Practical Thinking." In *The Culture of Craft: Status and Future*. Manchester and New York: Manchester University Press, pp. 137–57.

Fariello, M. Anna and Owen, Paula (eds). 2005. *Objects and Meaning: New Perspectives on Art and Craft*. Lanham, MD: The Scarecrow Press, Inc.

Field, Tiffany. 2001. *Touch*. Cambridge, MA: The MIT Press.

Hacker, Rose. 2007. "This Much I Know." April 1, *Observer Magazine*.

Heritage Studies Research Group. 2004. The Magic Touch: Touching and Handling in a Cultural Heritage Context (conference), Institute of Archaeology, University College London, December 20

Jerwood Charitable Foundation. 2008. *Jerwood Contemporary Makers* (catalogue). London: Jerwood Space.

Kemske, Bonnie. 2008. "Jerwood Contemporary Makers". *Ceramic Review*, 233 (September/October).

Lebovich, Jennifer. 2004. "Thousands Wait Hours for a Hug." *New York Daily News* (July 19). Cited in C. Classen (ed.) 2005, *The Book of Touch*. Oxford: Berg.

Light, Kathleen C., Grewen, Karen M., and Amico, Janet A. 2005. "More Frequent Partner Hugs and Higher Oxytocin Levels are Linked to Lower Blood Pressure and Heart Rate in Premenopausal Women." *Biological Psychology*, 69 (1): 5–21.

Lumley, Robert. 2004. *Arte Povera*. London: Tate Publishing.

Lusher, Adam. 2006. "It's a Tight Squeeze as British Reserve Meets the Cuddle Party." October 14. http://www.telegraph.co.uk/news/uknews/1531450/Its-a-tight-squeeze-as-British-reserve-meets-the-cuddle-party.html (accessed: April 12, 2009).

Merleau-Ponty, Maurice. 1962. *The Phenomenology of Perception*. Translated by Colin Smith. London: Routledge.

Merleau-Ponty, Maurice. 1968. *The Visible and the Invisible: Followed by Working Notes*. Translated by Alphonso Lingis. Evanston, IL: Northwestern University Press.

Merleau-Ponty, Maurice. 2004. *Maurice Merleau-Ponty: Basic Writings*. Edited by Thomas Baldwin. Routledge: London.

Montagu, Ashley. 1986. *Touching: The Human Significance of the Skin*, 3rd edn. New York: Harper & Row Publishers.

Nishida, Kitarō. 1990. *An Inquiry into the Good*. New Haven, CT: Yale University Press.

Nishida, Kitarō. 2007. *Zen no kenkyu*. Cited in "Nishida Kitarō," Encyclopædia Brittanica. http://www.britannica.com/eb/article-5292 (accessed: August 17, 2007).

Olausson, H., Lamarre, Y., Backlund, H., et al. 2002. "Unmyelinated Tactile Afferents Signal Touch and Project to Insular Cortex." *Nature Neuroscience*, 5 (9): 900–4.

Polanyi, Michael. 1958. *Personal Knowledge: Towards a Post-Critical Philosophy*. London: Routledge & Kegan Paul.

Sennett, Richard. 2008. *The Craftsman*. St Ives: Allen Lane (Penguin Books).

Sinclair, David. 1981. *Mechanisms of Cutaneous Sensation*. Oxford: Oxford University Press.

Spence, Charles. 2004. "A Multisensory Approach to Touch," paper presented at The Magic Touch: Touching and Handling in a Cultural Heritage Context, University College London, December 20.

University for the Creative Arts. 2008. Memory and Touch: An Exploration of Textural Communication (exhibition and conference). http://www.ucreative.ac.uk/index.cfm?articleid=18890 (accessed: March 18, 2009).

Vasseleu, Cathryn. 1998. *Textures of Light: Vision and Touch in Irigaray, Levinas and Merleau-Ponty*. London: Routledge.

Victoria and Albert Museum. 2005. Touch Me: Design and Sensation. Exhibition, London, June 16 to August 29. http://www.vam.ac.uk/vastatic/microsites/1376_touch_me/ (accessed: June 11, 2007).

DESIGN REVIEW

Senses & Society   VOLUME 4, ISSUE 3   REPRINTS AVAILABLE   PHOTOCOPYING   © BERG 2009
                     PP 347–352   DIRECTLY FROM THE   PERMITTED BY   PRINTED IN THE UK
                                            PUBLISHERS   LICENSE ONLY

The Heathcote School: An Object Lesson

Amy F. Ogata

Amy F. Ogata is Associate Professor at the Bard Graduate Center for Studies in the Decorative Arts, Design and Culture in New York City. She is currently preparing a book on creativity and the material culture of postwar American childhood.
ogata@bgc.bard.edu

When it opened in 1953, the Heathcote School was one of the most lavish and expensive public elementary schools built in the United States. Located in the wealthy New York City suburb of Scarsdale on a 22 acre site, the school plant sprawls across the rolling hilltop in a cluster plan of isolated pavilions connected by long glazed corridors to a central building with offices, art and music rooms, a shop room, and an auditorium. In plan and details, the school was designed to stimulate the senses and embodied the progressive concerns of postwar education to promote learning by engaging the child physically and psychologically.

Heathcote's architects, Lawrence B. Perkins and Philip Will of Perkins, Wheeler, Will of Chicago, were known for school buildings designed around progressive values of discovery, aesthetic appreciation, and a wholesome sense of security. Perkins and Will were the co-architects, with Eliel and Eero Saarinen, of the influential Crow Island School (1939–40) in Winnetka, Illinois, which became famous for its self-contained "home-like" classrooms with adjoining gardens, space for hands-on classroom projects, and

Senses & Society   DOI 10.2752/174589209X12464528171978

curricular objective to stimulate curiosity. Building on a nineteenth-century kindergarten tradition of learning through the senses, postwar public elementary schools in wealthy suburbs like Winnetka and Scarsdale adopted a progressive outlook to cultivate the individual and preserve their towns' upper-middle-class character. Scarsdale's Superintendent, Archibald B. Shaw, described the district's educational philosophy as "concern with the pupil – both as an individual and as a member of the group"(Shaw and Perkins 1954). The plan of the school therefore reinforces autonomy and community. Four hexagonal classrooms in each of the five clusters share a foyer area with coat racks and bathrooms that was also used for team teaching. The flower-shaped clusters, which the architects likened to "children under a tree," gently separate the grades and ages. Nearly circular in shape, the classrooms offered an open, radiant-heated floor area for multiple activities and directed children to focus on each other. The original moveable furniture reflected the school's desire for flexible instruction in small and large groups. Each

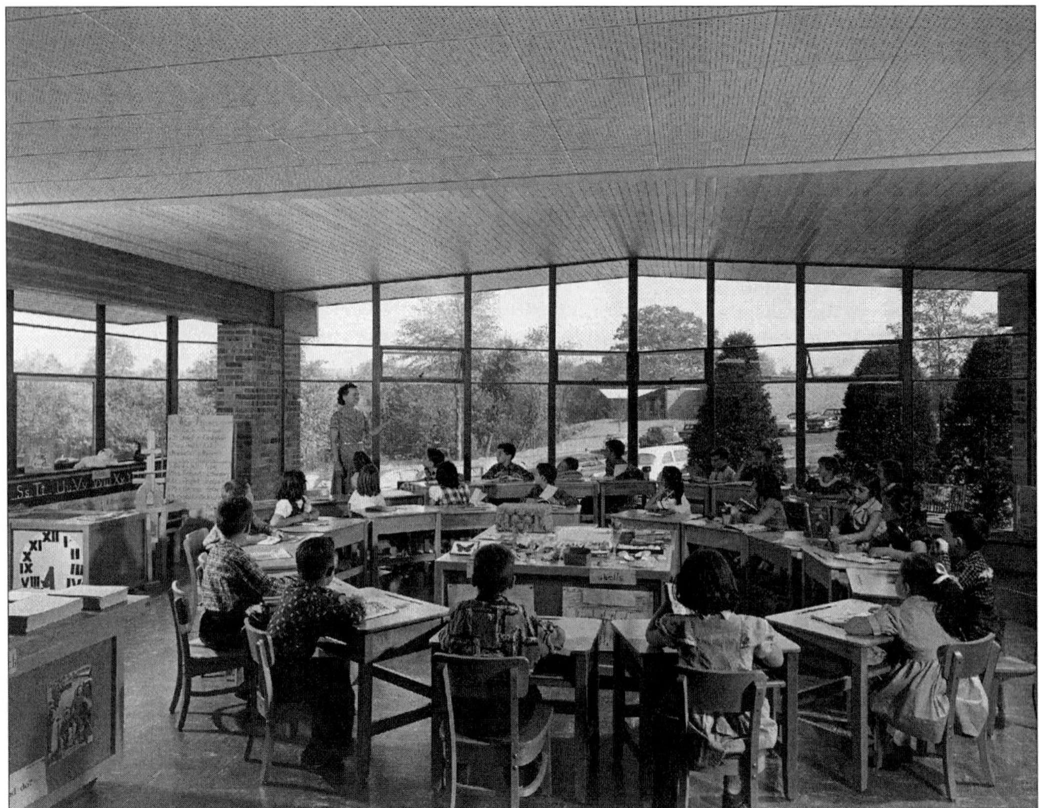

Figure 1
Classroom, Heathcote School, 1953. Photograph courtesy of Hedrich-Blessing, Chicago History Museum, HB16711-L.

classroom has two glass walls that reach from the ceiling to the low built-in seats, enhancing the child's awareness of the surrounding landscape. The extensive use of plate glass throughout the school constantly suggests spatial openness to the wooded terrain and provides visual contact with other students and teachers. Even the gymnasium has tall windows and shallow built-in benches on the perimeter, allowing light to flood the play area and views out to a courtyard.

The use of glass and color in the long hallways that follow the undulating topography is perhaps Heathcote's key feature. Unlike other schools of the period, the corridors are not open to weather, nor do they have a series of classrooms strung along them. Instead, Heathcote's halls are glazed on both sides and inset with brilliant jewel-colored glass panes placed at various heights, casting a bright grid on the linoleum floors and inviting children, and adults, to gaze through and rediscover the surrounding landscape in orange, blue, or green. Similar panes once adorned a wall in the Kindergarten

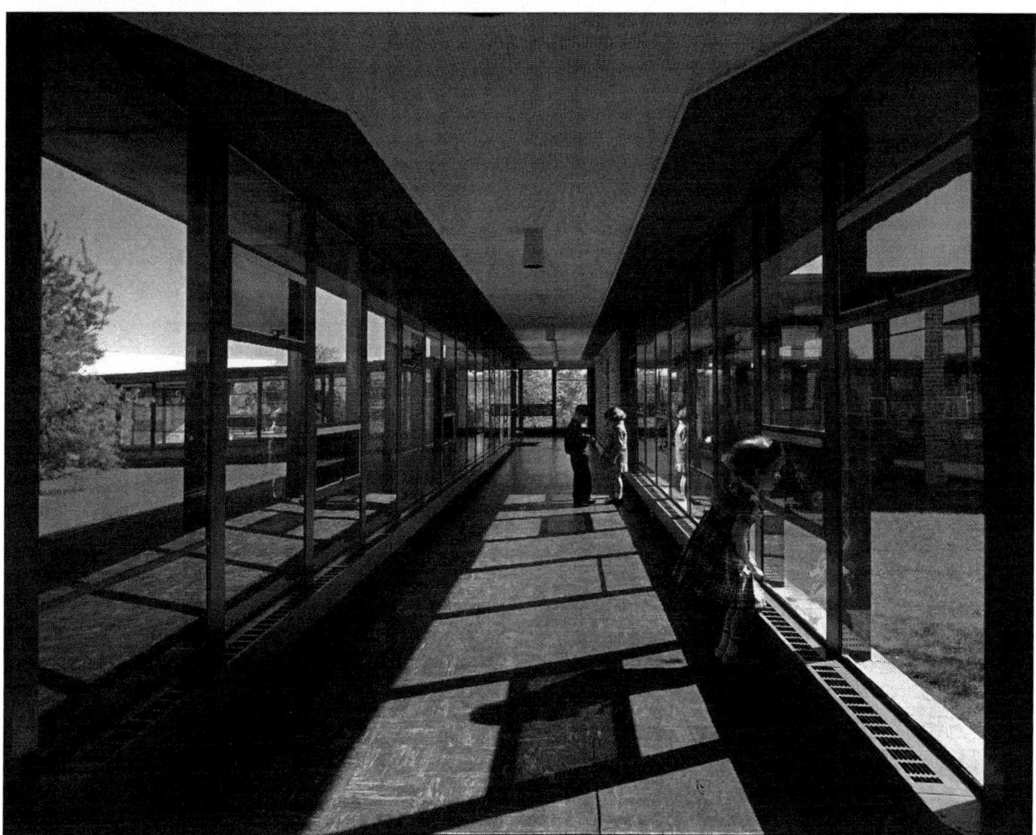

Figure 2
Hallway, Heathcote School, 1953. Photograph courtesy of Hedrich-Blessing, Chicago History Museum, HB-1611-X.

playroom along with brightly tiled bathrooms. These spots of vivid color added interest to the building's relatively neutral palette of varnished wood and brick, and were included expressly to engage the pupils' senses. As prominent American school architects noted in 1951, "the sensation of colour may create feelings of pleasantness and harmony, of drabness and depression, or of stimulation and excitability. It is just this factor which causes colour to be of such importance in the classroom, for the classroom is the home – the environment – of the learning process" (Caudill and Pena 1951: 123).

The Perkins and Will firm made their name designing schools that deliberately eschewed a cold institutional image in favor of intimate buildings constructed to reassure and please children. The architects were keenly aware of the psychological research of the period, which suggested that young children often felt overwhelmed in large spaces. Following the domestic architecture of the era, the firm stressed single-story construction, and used lower ceilings, deep overhanging roofs, and expansive glass windows. The prominent rooflines and large chimney – the hearth being one of Perkins and Will's signature forms – dominate Heathcote's low-rise profile and put it in context with the single-family housing nearby. While the ceiling heights in the public areas are low, they rise in the center of the hexagonal classrooms, and in the gymnasium and auditorium. Furthermore, the low-pitch roofs at Heathcote extend well beyond the glass walls, producing an overwhelming sense of shelter. Deliberately evoking the informality of home, the library has multiple levels, including a sunken area with windows, built-in brick planters, and a fireplace, in front of which children were encouraged to read sprawling comfortably on colorful cushions.

Throughout the school, Perkins and Will juxtaposed contrasting materials, spatial volumes, and experiences. The auditorium is sited prominently near the front of the school as an emblem of community, its semi-circular brick walls and deep rounded stage rephrasing the geometry of the individual classrooms. Since the stage is pushed into the seating area, the auditorium is intimate and designed acoustically to capture the voices of small children. The expanses of smooth glass that reach into the site hug the open grounds and a large play area, which still has some original equipment. In addition to swings, there are three tubular steel climbing arches and a cast concrete turtle, part of a series of "Play Sculpture" produced by the postwar educational toy firm Creative Playthings, Inc. Along with the noisy open play yard, there is an interior courtyard for quiet contemplation that includes a landscaped area with large rocks for climbing and sitting, which was originally paved with rough stones for occasional outdoor instruction. Heathcote was designed for children to look, touch and hear in spaces scaled for them, to encourage reflection and participation, security and exploration.

Heathcote was one of thousands of new schools built after World War II to meet the growing needs of the baby boom in the United

States. Many architects embraced the low-rise model, experimented with efficient steel-frame construction, used vast amounts of glass in their buildings, and acknowledged the importance of the child's experience (Ogata 2008). "School plant architecture," according to a handbook written by a prominent planner and architect, "must recognize that its forms, dimensions, color, materials, and texture are capable of creating an environment which either attracts or repels the child" (Bursch and Reid 1947: 6). Yet few school districts across the country could afford to invest in the tactile, aural, and visual pleasures of Heathcote. Although it was built in an era of rising technical standards – when other architects were diligently measuring classroom luminosity and optimal air circulation to improve posture and attention – Perkins noted emphatically that Heathcote rejected "the current concentration on how to pour air over a child, throw light on his book, fit his contours to the seats. This building is not an exercise in lighting and ventilation." Instead, he claimed to focus on "the in'ards of the child" (*Architectural Forum* 1952: 114). Heathcote belongs to a concurrent discourse in progressive circles that the color, sound, and feeling of materials, space, and the natural landscape could engage pupils' senses and focus their own subjective experience. At the same time, however, it was an unusually complex and refined statement of these postwar values.

Even as the building has aged, it retains much, if not all, of its original character. Additions, beginning in 1958 with the completion of the fifth cluster of classrooms, and subtle adjustments to room usage (the computer lab was once the shop room) have had a minor effect on the school's overall appearance. In other ways, however, the sensory experience for which the school was justly renown has changed. Although trees and grass were planted near the plate-glass walls to combat glare in the classrooms, blinds have been added to the brightest exposures, and larger seating and case furniture (there is little provision for storage) interrupts the openness of the classroom floor. Furthermore, the number of colored glass panes in the corridors is greatly reduced and the addition of handrails obstructs one of the few remaining low-placed panes. The broader object lessons of the Heathcote School are nonetheless intact. Built in an age of Cold War anxieties to serve a rapidly expanding population, Heathcote's designers (architects, school board officials, local citizens, and teachers) envisioned an institution that would entice children to learn not only in, but also from their environment.

References

Bursch, Charles Wesley and Reid, John Lyon. 1947. *You Want to Build a School?* New York: Reinhold.

Caudill, W.W. and Pena, W.M. 1951. "Colour in the Classroom." *Journal of Royal Architectural Institute of Canada* May: 123.

Architectural Forum. 1952. "Organic School: Humanist Approach Yields Bold New Ideas for Classrooms and Auditorium," October: 114.

Ogata, Amy F. 2008. "Building for Learning in Postwar American Elementary Schools." *Journal of the Society of Architectural Historians* 67(4): 562–91.
Shaw, Archibald B. and Perkins, Lawrence B. 1954. "Planning an Elementary School." *School Executive* July (73): 59.

BOOK REVIEWS

Senses & Society   **VOLUME 4, ISSUE 3**   **REPRINTS AVAILABLE**   **PHOTOCOPYING**   © BERG 2009
           PP 355–358   **DIRECTLY FROM THE**   **PERMITTED BY**   PRINTED IN THE UK
                    PUBLISHERS   **LICENSE ONLY**

Selective Sensory Environments: Changing Experiences of Public Life through City Regeneration Practices

Sensing Cities: Regenerating Public Life in Barcelona and Manchester, by Mónica Montserrat Degen

London and New York: Routledge,
Taylor & Francis Group, 2008, 225 pp.
HB 978-0-415-39799-5. £75.00/$150.00.

Victoria Henshaw and Mags Adams

Victoria Henshaw is a doctoral candidate in the Built and Human Environment at the University of Salford, UK, and is Chair of the Doncaster Design and Architecture Centre situated in the North of England.
v.henshaw@pgr.salford.ac.uk

Mags Adams is a Senior Research Fellow in the Acoustics Research Centre and Research Institute of the Built and Human Environment, University of Salford, UK, and recently convened the ESRC research seminar series "Rethinking the urban experience: the sensory production of place."
m.d.adams@salford.ac.uk

The public life of cities as experienced through the bodies of those who reside, carry out business, travel through or appropriate space in the course of other sanctioned or illicit activity poses a complex

Senses & Society DOI 10.2752/174589209X12464528172012

research challenge, further complicated by the added necessity to investigate the experiences of those excluded from, or choosing to avoid, such spaces. It is this that Mónica Degen sets out to explore and elucidate in her captivating account of the changing urban environments brought about by regeneration activity in two European city districts.

Mónica Degen's *Sensing Cities* offers an enjoyable, perceptive, comparative analysis between Castlefield, an area targeted as the site for the delivery of Britain's first Urban Heritage Park in the 1980s, and El Ravel, Barcelona's historically marginal and increasingly ethnically diverse district, also home to the internationally celebrated Museum of Contemporary Art of Barcelona (MACBA), opened in 1995.

Although markedly different in culture, urban form, and levels of existing public life, both areas are experiencing the effects of global commercial forces at a local level. They are targeted for regeneration activity specifically designed to parade an idealized cosmopolitan image of the districts and their respective cities on what Degen terms "the Global Catwalk" for investment and tourism. As such, the two sites are ideal candidates for examining Degen's key concern of understanding how modern-day regeneration processes are transforming the sensory qualities of place, and whether the resulting sensory reorganization has the effect of excluding or including particular cultural expressions and practices in the public life of these areas and the spaces created within them. Paradoxically, it is herein that our only real criticism of this book lies: the two sites selected for comparison are located in so called "postindustrial" European cities, and as such the findings are reflective of regeneration practices within such cities. Degen might therefore have further developed her thoughts through exploring and discussing, if to a much lesser degree, the relationship between her findings and the experiences of sites in smaller towns or cities that might have different relationships with consumption potentially targeting regeneration activity and related city marketing strategies at an alternative point in the competitive hierarchy, be it at a regional or national level.

Notwithstanding this minor criticism, the book is full of revealing examples and insights into sensory assumptions, motivations, and practices ingrained within modern-day city development and globally targeted regeneration practices, and it provides a welcome and useful contribution to the burgeoning body of literature on the sensory experiences of urban environments. It provides a useful resource for built environment professionals and academics alike and investigates and illustrates the impacts these can have on the public life of areas targeted for regeneration – whether as a planned or unforeseen consequence.

The book draws on Degen's own empirical research carried out in Castlefield and El Ravel between 1997 and 2002, bringing together observations and further developing arguments made within her previous writings on sensory environments and related public life.

Following a logical and accessible format structured into two broad sections, Degen commences by building her arguments through a discussion of literature on public life in later modernity, sensuous cities, power, and planning ideologies that focus primarily on the visual. Drawing strongly on the writings of Lefebvre, who suggests that spaces are socially produced and experienced through a sensuous body, Degen develops a theoretical tool of "socially embedded aesthetics" of place that allows corporeal analysis through capturing the ways in which daily embodied sensory experience and the social character of the senses organize the "publicness" of spaces.

In the second section of the book, Degen presents the background to each area, describing the historical, social, and economic environments of Castlefield and El Ravel, and in doing so identifies characteristics inherent within many traditionally poorer, working-class, and industrial urban areas across the globe. These characteristics bring with them highly sensory environments and associations, including provision of residential accommodation for poorer and immigrant communities, marginal and undesirable activities such as prostitution and drug abuse, and the location of dirty and polluting industrial trades and premises. Additionally, facilities that were perceived by the bourgeoisie as a risk to public health were also located in these areas, including hospitals and children's homes. Degen's description culminates with an outline of the physical, social, and organizational environment experienced at the turn of the millennium in the two areas, including a focus upon the activities and physical restructuring leading up to the delivery of flagship projects and public space in the two respective areas – the Castlefield Events Arena in Manchester and MACBA in Barcelona.

Degen analyses and discusses the publicness of these urban spaces through applying her concept of socially embedded aesthetics. She is successful in this through structuring her thoughts around Lefebvre's interrelated trialectic – conceived space (how representations of space inform conceptions of how public a space should be), perceived space (the observable configurations and behavior within space), and the actual lived experience of space. Furthermore, Degen draws from Lefebvre's rhythmanalysis, as a method which involves the observation through a variety of sensoria of the activity and sensory mapping of a landscape, in order to assess the perceived and actual lived experiences of space.

By structuring her analysis in this way, Degen successfully illustrates the motivations behind the regeneration activities in both Castlefield and El Ravel alongside the various planning and development paradigms upon which these are based. In both cases, and somewhat unsurprisingly, regeneration is shown to have been implemented with the aim of enhancing the global appeal of the cities in which they are situated through the standardization and control of urban life. In Castlefield, however, this was led by a desire to deliver new formalized public spaces and a new form of public life for the city, whilst in El Ravel it was aimed at assimilating the district into the wider city whole thus diluting existing public life in the area. Although these short-term planning goals are identified as having been successfully delivered, Degen goes on to argue that the changes brought about by regeneration activities are lived experiences understood through the body, and thus by focusing upon the senses during periods of urban change it is possible to illustrate the complex nature of urban space and its relationship to public life. The interaction of local and global processes exposed as a result, such as the tendency for such spaces to support the segregation of diverse publics and activities, resulting in the existence of parallel public lives, is argued to be creating new forms of spatial contest that threaten the long-term social cohesion of the city.

A well-researched and well-written publication, *Sensing Cities* offers a fascinating and accessible account of this complex and extremely topical subject matter, building upon the classic sensory theories of Sennett and Lefebvre, and sitting well in a contemporary genre of work including that of authors such as Howes, Urry, and Edensor. The insights offered by Degen are guaranteed to resonate with all readers, stimulating further discussion and research on sensory environmental experience and locality, power structures and decision-making processes, and their complex interplay in the form in which public life in cities is experienced.

Senses & Society   VOLUME 4, ISSUE 3   **REPRINTS AVAILABLE**   **PHOTOCOPYING**   © BERG 2009
PP 359–362   **DIRECTLY FROM THE**   **PERMITTED BY**   PRINTED IN THE UK
PUBLISHERS   **LICENSE ONLY**

Sensing Dance

Sensational Knowledge: Embodying Culture through Japanese Dance, by Tomie Hahn

Middletown, Connecticut: Wesleyan
University Press, 2007, 224 pp.
DVD 6 × 9". PB 978-0-8195-6835-9. $26.95,
HB 978-0-8195-6834-2. $70.00.

Sally Ann Ness

**Sally Ann Ness is
Professor of Anthropology
at the University of
California, Riverside,
author of Body,
Movement, and Culture
(1992), and co-editor of
Migrations of Gesture
(2008). Her research
has focused on various
forms of symbolic
action observable
in choreographic
phenomena. She is
currently focusing on
touristic forms of motility
practiced and performed
in Yosemite National Park.
sally.ness@ucr.edu.**

"Transmission" is currently orienting a new wave of research in performance studies, serving as a conceptual platform for attempts to find more fluid ways to reconfigure agency and subjecthood in the wake of globalization. Tomie Hahn's study of the Japanese dance genre *nihon buyo* finds a place within this movement. While Hahn's focus on how nihon buyo is passed down from one generation to the next is something like the converse of the typical globalization project – foregrounding, as it does, continuities of pedagogy that perpetuate tradition – the way in which performing subjects are observed as vehicles of the culture that is considered to "flow" within the practice is very much in line with the larger wave of research.

Hahn's strategy for understanding how cultural transmission occurs in nihon buyo centers on the observation of

Senses & Society   DOI 10.2752/174589209X12464528172058

"the senses" (p. 2). The senses are posited as the interface between bodies, selves, and the nihon buyo world of teaching/learning. Positioning herself as following in the footsteps of scholars she identifies as already having bridged the mind–body divide (Barbara Browning and Cynthia Bull), Hahn states that she intends, through sensory examination, to offer the reader a way to "know with the body" (p. 8) in a manner that reveals how a social group can come to share "experiential orientations" and interactive "structures" (p. 5) basic to cultural practice.

The core of the text is the seventy-four-page Chapter Four, "Revealing Lessons." It is placed after two shorter chapters that sketch the history of nihon buyo in relation to traditional Japanese performing arts and summarize its key stylistic components. In Chapter Four, Hahn identifies and exemplifies the knowledge she observes embodied through visual, tactile, and oral/aural sensory modes of transmission. The chapter is designed to be read in tandem with a DVD that accompanies the text, and provides examples of each mode. A final brief section also discusses media-based forms of transmission (notation and video) which Hahn observes playing only a marginal role in the teaching of the practice to date.

The interlacing of the DVD and the written text is intricate, to the extent that Chapter Four cannot stand alone as an independent essay. In describing "visual transmission," (p. 81) for example, Hahn analyzes three dance lessons partially documented on the DVD, observing strategies used in each by students attempting to follow the teacher through a segment of choreography. A fourth DVD example is provided for the reader's own "orienting" exercise, one of several Hahn includes throughout the text to allow readers to participate bodily in transmission processes. The degree of text/DVD coupling represents a new type of media integration in culturally focused dance analysis. At times the text reads as an extended caption for the DVD examples; at times it verges on a how-to discourse, but at others it achieves a kind of descriptive *experience* that places the reader in the middle of a scene of unfolding movement in a strikingly original manner. Hahn's experimental efforts in this regard are generative, although unevenly so. However, the unevenness is, perhaps, an indicator of the novelty of the interactive learning she attempts to reveal and develop.

In the final chapter, "Transforming Sensu," Hahn focuses on trans-figuration, drawing on the sociolinguistic concept of code-switching. The continual dis-/reorienting experiences of code-switching acts that occur in the performance of multiple character roles, Hahn argues, enable dancers to know with their bodies a wider range of cultural identities through nihon buyo than would otherwise be accessible to them. The notion of code-switching allows Hahn to link dance practice to a much wider domain of cultural meaning-making than her sensory approach otherwise might do, drawing parallels between nihon buyo and the linguistic practices of Japanese life, everyday and extraordinary. It leads her as well into a discussion of "presence," the galvanizing synthesis that transforms a dancer's studied demonstrations into unfolding works of art when they "put it all together" (p. 163) in performance. Hahn's recognition that such presence is in fact *transmittable* constitutes a provocative theoretical move, challenging assumptions about the ephemerality of performance that have gone largely unchecked in theoretical discourses until recently. While Hahn's appeal to linguistic theory in this final chapter comes as a surprise, given the sensorial orientation of her project, the conceptual shift is productive.

Hahn relies on more than thirty years of experience dancing nihon buyo to ground her study. Her practical understanding often seems to override her sensory theory in ways that significantly enrich her descriptive project. The best example of this is found in her account of her *sensu*, her fan, which she uses as a trope for structuring the text as a whole. Hahn never puts the reader through a multisensory analysis of her sensu practice. Instead, she uses imagery, metaphor, and narratives of performance to sketch the living role the sensu plays as her partner in dancing. The effect is compelling, opening up the world Hahn inhabits in performance vividly and concretely. Even when following "the senses," however, Hahn's practice-based orientation leads to a recognition of how sensation rarely, if ever, divides into processes occurring in isolated sense organs – as the text's organization would suggest. In Chapter Four's segment on aural/oral sensing, for example, Hahn describes how the sensing of sound entails not only the use of the ears but the movement of the whole body, including the eyes. Rather than looking separately at "each" sense, Hahn's descriptions more typically foreground distinctive patterns of sensory integration that orient culturally specific experiences of movement.

Hahn's insightful practitioner identity comes at a price, however. In this regard, her work resembles greatly, both in its strengths and its weaknesses, that of her scholarly ancestor, Cynthia Bull. As in Bull's now-classic research on American contact improvisational dance, the spirit of near-absolute deference for the community that bears the culture embodied at times overwhelms the ability to observe the totality of its cultural predicament critically. Asymmetries of power both within the practice and outside it are off the analytical table with very few exceptions. While Hahn cannot avoid recognizing the racism, sexism, and elitism embedded in nihon buyo's cultural context, the perspective she takes on its practices of cultural transmission has a somewhat utopian character. The picture that emerges seems incomplete, although not necessarily inaccurate as far as it goes.

On the positive side, the reverence with which Hahn approaches her subject yields a poignant authorial voice that readers, particularly students, will find appealing and admirable. *Sensational Knowledge* is an exceptionally good book for use in teaching, raising important issues of both method and theory about the relationship between embodiment and culture. If its sometimes disorienting conceptual shifts leave big questions unanswered – particularly the question of how far down into the human biological organism "culture" can go through its sensory transmissions – the carefully attuned account of nihon buyo training processes situates these slippages within a vivid world of practice, configuring them as invitations rather than barriers to greater understanding.

Senses & Society   VOLUME 4, ISSUE 3   REPRINTS AVAILABLE   PHOTOCOPYING   © BERG 2009
PP 363–366   DIRECTLY FROM THE   PERMITTED BY   PRINTED IN THE UK
PUBLISHERS   LICENSE ONLY

Touchy Subjects

The Senses of Touch: Haptics, Affects and Technologies, by Mark Paterson

Oxford and New York: Berg, 2007, 224 pp.
PB 978-1-845-20479-2. $34.95.

The Politics of Touch: Sense, Movement, Sovereignty, by Erin Manning

Minneapolis: University of Minnesota Press, 2006, 195 pp. PB 978-0-816-64845-0. $22.50.

Carrie Purcell

Carrie Purcell is a PhD student in the Sociology Department at the University of Edinburgh whose doctoral research looks at touch and embodiment in the context of holistic massage work. Based on her masters' research, she has also published on the experience of male therapeutic massage workers.
c.a.purcell@sms.ed.ac.uk

One of the most interesting facets of touch and of the senses more generally is that they are open to investigation from a variety of disciplinary perspectives, and this interdisciplinarity is well represented by the two books reviewed here. Both Mark Paterson and Erin Manning combine perspectives from classical and contemporary philosophy, anthropology, sociology, the natural sciences, engineering, and the arts to offer

Senses & Society   DOI 10.2752/174589209X12464528172094

rich explorations of touch and its metaphors. My own primarily sociological interest in touch having developed fairly recently, I was enthused to see such diversity in approaches.

Paterson's pluralizing of *The Senses of Touch* in the title of the book is significant in indicating the author's approach to these senses as both multiple and varied, and the book excels in considering these different areas. The glossary provided at the front is particularly useful in specifying the precise meaning of terms employed, particularly given the variation across texts in the use, for example, of *tactile* and *haptic*. Beyond the glossary the book is compiled of eight chapters structured so as to work inwards from the more literal, superficial aspects of touch towards deeper metaphorical associations, and while it is a fascinating cover-to-cover read, chapters may also be dipped into individually.

Chapter 1, "The Primacy of Touch," begins with an exploration of the philosophical roots of Western understandings of touch and goes on to invert the Aristotelian hierarchy of the senses, situating touch rather than vision as prime. The chapter also introduces the chief concerns of the volume such as challenging the "ocularcentrism" (a term borrowed from Martin Jay) of contemporary society, the interplay between touch and vision. Having led the reader from ancient Greek sensual constructions to the Christian tradition, the author moves on to (relatively) more recent philosophical approaches, primarily the phenomenology of Merleau-Ponty. In Chapter 2 Paterson develops the key conceptual framework of a "felt phenomenology," which brings together phenomenological theory with what might be termed a holistic approach to the bodily senses, and then explores how such a framework may be used to "articulate" the multiple senses of touch. Phenomenology is proposed and justified as an appropriate means of approaching the senses given the attention to lived embodiment in the work not only of Husserl and Merleau-Ponty but others such as Alfred Schutz. It is this *felt* phenomenology which the author goes on to explore in subsequent chapters.

The third chapter, which appeared as an article in an earlier issue of this journal, focuses on Paterson's obviously keen interest in the relationship between the senses. Bringing together philosophy and neuroscience, the interplay between vision, touch, and under-standings of space are examined in the case of both sighted and blind experience (the philosophical fascination with blindness is to be expanded upon in a forthcoming title from the author). Here the author notes the predominance of a Cartesian model of touch as "seeing with the hands," which situates the latter as inferior in relation to sight. The following chapter turns to geometry, and while I found this to be the driest of the eight, it successfully highlights the shift in a once fully embodied discipline which has become somewhat impoverished through its reduction to abstract notations. Paterson poses the question of how the "embodied process of measuring actual multidimensional spaces become abstracted into two-dimensional symbols and relations" (p. 60), a question relevant to much social science methodology.

The fifth and sixth chapters attend to "haptic aesthetics." Chapter 5 considers examples of painting, sculpture, and architecture and Chapter 6 uses Deleuze's notion of the *fold* as a narrative device employed to lead the reader through the layers of *skin*, *flesh*, and *body* as well as addressing the work of body artists such as Orlan and Stelarc. Where the examples presented in each chapter are somewhat removed from everyday life, they are – particularly in "Tangible Play" – successfully, carnally presented as means for thinking through the body. Chapter 7, "Technologies of Touch," examines the significance of new technologies of touch, from the relatively ubiquitous iPod, to more specialist tools developed from the PHANToM haptic device – first built at MIT in the early 1990s – and the ways in which these collapse distance and allow the sensing of presence and co-presence. The creation of co-presence or proximity is drawn out as a primary aim in the development of such innovation, a theme which continues into the final chapter.

"Affecting Touch: Flesh and Feeling-With" was the chapter I expected to be the most interesting, both for its empirical focus on therapeutic touching and its attention to affect and the blurred boundary between touching and feeling. Given the considerable history of the use of touch as a therapeutic means, to suggest that it was at one stage "unorthodox" is somewhat misleading, and the promise of empirical engagement with therapeutic touching was also rather disappointing, as Paterson's exploration of Reiki in the end amounts to less than half a dozen pages. However, the conclusion that the creation of physical and/or emotional proximity is one of the most significant aspects of this phenomenon is a crucial one which deserves further attention. Paterson returns to the problems of the gap between articulating touch through the medium of language versus the immediacy of feeling in this final chapter, and his approach certainly takes a step towards narrowing this gap. A thought-provoking book on the whole, *The Senses of Touch* will be of use to those with an interest in bodies, senses, and haptics (in the broad sense used by Paterson), and would be most accessible to a postgraduate audience onwards.

Erin Manning's *The Politics of Touch: Sense, Movement, Sovereignty* is a challenging text in a number of ways. Over its introduction and six chapters it offers various "lines of flight" which I found to be more focused on space and movement than on touch *per se*. Manning clearly intends to mount a challenge to conventional political–philosophical thinking about bodies and senses, in particular through the concept established, in the introduction, of the body as a "sensing body in movement," rather than the fixed, stable entity that political systems would apparently have us believe. Tango, which is utilized as an effective and evocative refrain throughout the book, is attended to in greatest detail in the first chapter, in which it is posited as an example of a "politics of touch." Here, Manning considers the literal and linguistic associations of *tango* alongside the social history of the dance and its fluid, shifting character, ultimately characterizing both tango and touch as a "reaching towards," a creation of space through movement.

Chapter 2 continues with the tango leitmotif via an examination of Wong Kar Wai's 1997 film *Happy Together*, which the author frames as being about "two bodies seeking sensation" (p. 19), a search which propels them in and out of their various relationships. The chapter offers an insightful reading of the film (some rather grating references to "Asians" and "homosexuals" aside) in which the focus on spatiality continues, with friendship, for example, being described as "the space between friends." Several stills from the film are also included, although their quality as reproduced does little to convey Wong's signature visual style and therefore they add little to the chapter.

The third chapter, "Erring Towards Experience: Violence and Touch," is the longest of the six and provides a (re-)examination of touching metaphors in the Bible. The act of original sin is re-framed as a touching act, and the *noli me tangere* episode (Jesus's words to Mary Magdalene when she recognised him after his resurrection as reported in the Gospel of John) is considered as a means of highlighting the opposition of touch and the "corporeal presence" it requires, with faith and the willingness to believe without the option of feeling for the truth. Chapter 4, "Engenderings: Gender, Politics, Individuation," draws primarily on Butler, and among other issues refers to problems tied to expressing touch, which "exceeds language's significability" (a concern shared not only by Paterson, but by anyone involved in touch scholarship). The penultimate chapter, "Making Sense of the Incommensurable," offers an interesting exploration of skin and its ephemeral nature, and Chapter 6, "Sensing beyond Security," focuses on the Deluzian *body without organs*, including an engaging discussion of the literal and metaphorical association between touch and tact.

Manning's argument is willfully non-linear, looping this way and that, which enhances an overall sense of movement within the text and is in keeping with the tango refrain. However, while the author is thus successful in creating a dynamic text, I found the book to be frustrating to say the least. Where Paterson challenges the reader to embody the methodological approach he proposes, Manning evokes a feeling of distance from the bodies that lie at the heart of politics and of touch, an intangibility which I found ultimately unsatisfying. Frustrations aside, this volume is worth reading for the eclectic sources drawn on and the proposed re-formulation of the senses for politics, but may perhaps be of most interest to a specialist audience.

Senses & Society VOLUME 4, ISSUE 3 REPRINTS AVAILABLE PHOTOCOPYING © BERG 2009
PP 367–372 DIRECTLY FROM THE PERMITTED BY PRINTED IN THE UK
PUBLISHERS LICENSE ONLY

Theory and Practice: The Senses in the Middle Ages

Rethinking the Medieval Senses: Heritage, Fascinations, Frames, by Stephen G. Nichols, Andreas Kablitz and Alison Calhoun (eds)

Baltimore, MD: The Johns Hopkins University Press, 2008. xii, 327 pp. PB 978-0-8018-8737-6: $24.95; HB 978-0-8018-8736-9: $65

The Senses in Late Medieval England, by C. M. Woolgar

New Haven, CT and London: Yale University Press, 2006. xii, 372 pp. HB 0-300-11871-6: $40

Richard G. Newhauser

Richard G. Newhauser is a professor of English at Arizona State University, Tempe, specializing in Middle English literature and intellectual history. richard.newhauser@asu.edu

Medieval Studies have come with some delay, but with full engagement, to their senses. The study of the sensorium in other historical periods has of late attracted increasing attention in various disciplines

Senses & Society DOI 10.2752/174589209X12500073929205

within the humanities. However, for a number of reasons having to do in part with the alterity of sensory information transmitted by medieval texts and partially with the denigration of sensory perception in many theological works in the Middle Ages, medieval scholars have only relatively recently joined in the undertaking of sensology. Two new and important publications provide insight into the directions of this current research on the functions of the sensorium in the material and intellectual cultures of the Middle Ages.

The collection of essays edited by Nichols *et al.* is the fruit of cooperation between historians and literary scholars (mainly in the Romance languages) at American and European universities. It is divided into four sections: on philosophical conceptualizations of the senses, their literary representations, and particular cultural and historical contexts of the medieval sensorium. In the first section, Eugene Vance focuses on Augustine of Hippo's view of the physiology of sensation and the role of the inner sense as a control mechanism of perception. In keeping with his Neoplatonist orientation, Augustine understood this process working in two directions: mental acts provoke the inner sense "to somatize the life of the mind" (p. 20), but the inner sense also receives and organizes corporeal sensation to make it useful for the soul. Gregor Vogt-Spira, emphasizing the Aristotelian tradition, demonstrates the epistemological dependence of thought on sensation in this tradition: for Aristotle and his interpreters through the early modern period, without sensation there can be no thought (p. 51). One consequence of this model of the soul for literary creation was to emphasize the role of imagination (*phantasia*), which allowed sense perception in the realm of reality to become equivalent to the action of the imagination evoked by texts. In a far-reaching essay based on Greek, Arabic and Latin works, Daniel Heller-Roazen presents a concise view of the early history of common sense, not as a type of comprehension shared by all humanity, but as a perceptive power that ranks as one of the primary faculties of the soul (p. 32). For Aristotle, common sense perceived common sensibles, but it also amounted to the perception of perception itself. Commentators in later centuries interpreted this variously: Isaac Israeli made of common sense the point at which each sense fades into the next, Avicenna understood it to be the imaginative faculty, Albert the Great developed Avicenna's idea to arrive at a view of common sense as a power which produces and contains within itself all of the senses proper.

Section two is devoted to reflexes of the senses in literature. Marina Brownlee extends the "oral sense" beyond eating, drinking and speech to include laughter, using this category to examine the dissonance in expected patterns of perception and cognition in two Spanish texts of the early fourteenth century. In the way the senses prove unreliable in some *exempla* in *Zifar* and *Lucanor*, she finds evidence of the increasing traction of Nominalist skepticism and considerations of human agency and subjectivity in this period

(p. 78). Michel Zink's meditation on the *locus amoenus* focuses on the way in which the senses are saturated in this site of endless pleasures, but humanity is also reminded of being subject to the laws of nature, which means the potential of change on the one hand and generation (love) on the other. The poetry of Boethius, William IX of Aquitaine and Matthew of Vêndome document the interplay between the four elements and the five senses. Variations in the hierarchy of sight and hearing in ancient and medieval epiphanies are the subject of Rainer Warning's contribution. In writing to Beatrice, Warning notes, Dante continues the dominance of word over vision in reports of epiphany inherited from Christian scriptures, but here epiphany is effected by its literary representation, not the intervention of divinity, and this deconstruction itself is thematized in Petrarch's response to Dante.

In section three, the cultural subtexts of the sensorium in ethics, politics, Salvation history and visuality are the focus. Using the example of Alfonso Martínez of Toledo's *Arcipreste de Talavera* (1438), Joachim Küpper's important essay examines the ethical implications of an essential paradox of the medieval senses (though Gabrielle Spiegel's comment on some of the essays in the volume queries whether this is dualism or paradox): epistemology is based on sensory perception, while Christian metaphysics demand a denunciation of the senses (p. 124). This contradiction provides an opening to the moral context of the sensorium in the Middle Ages, which describes the connection of the senses and volition. But Küpper finds here an impasse that cannot be perfected, arguing that if the means of perception are also the agents undermining cognition, the connection of perception and the will can have no coherence. David Nirenberg points to the homologous discourses of hermeneutics and political theory in which, he argues, the presence of the Jew was central throughout the Middle Ages. This "corporeal" Jewish status typified a type of "judaized" reading (adhering to the literal level and rejecting the spiritual), as it also characterized both aspirations to sovereignty (when a ruler claimed sole control of the Jews' fate in his realm) and political critique of some sovereigns for "royal judaizing." The last three essays deal with literary representations in mystery plays (Andreas Kablitz) and courtly epic (Jan-Dirk Müller, Hildegard Elisabeth Keller). Müller's essay deals with the way Konrad of Würzburg (second half of the thirteenth century) deconstructs the courtly paradigm of visuality in his *Trojanerkrieg*. Instead of sight yielding the truth of the court's aesthetic beauty, appearances prove deceptive and courtliness itself, without losing its luster, is revealed as potentially destructive. Using twelfth-century narratives of Ywain by Chrétien de Troyes and Hartmann von Aue, as well as frescoes in Schloss Rodenegg, Keller examines how the lack of visual perception—invisibility—is deployed in representing combat so that observers both in and outside the text achieve a bemused sovereignty over those who cannot see.

The last section treats the integration of realms often thought of now as separate: physiology and spirituality (Heather Webb); optics and literature (Stephen Nichols). Webb describes a discrete moment of "cardiosensory" (p. 266) assimilation in the late thirteenth and fourteenth centuries in which the integration of Aristotelian and Galenic ideas effected by Avicenna yielded a model of a life-process centered in the heart—both a physical organ and the seat of the soul. Perception by the five external senses, each of which is described here, was also understood as part of a unified physiological and spiritual process. Nichols emphasizes how the interest seen in images in the thirteenth-century *Romance of the Rose* and its many illuminated manuscripts are in harmony with Perspectivist optics developed from Arabic and Greek models. In Roger Bacon's *Perspectiva*, in particular, Nichols points to a text that constructed vision in the unified discourse of optics and theology that is characteristic of this period. As a whole, the collection of essays emphasizes the theoretical understanding of the senses—including the inner sense and sensuality altogether—in systematic treatments, many of which remain particular to the Middle Ages. As such, it is an invaluable statement of the importance of the sensorium in medieval intellectual history.

If the essay collection is focused on theoretical understandings of medieval sensation, Christopher Woolgar's monograph emphasizes the place of the senses in medieval practice. Though he makes mention of such theoretical issues as the internal senses (pp. 17–19), his book is centered on the five external senses. The study has two parts: ideas of the senses, which includes a detailed look at each one (dividing the senses of the mouth appropriately into taste and speech); and the everyday reality of the senses in the elite culture (bishops, queens and great households) of medieval England from the mid-twelfth to the mid-sixteenth century. The book is superbly printed on glossy paper with 86 color and black-and-white illustrations.

Even in the section on ideas of the senses, Woolgar is most interested in the day-to-day practicalities of sensation. His work is, in fact, a storehouse of detailed information on the cultural practice of sensation in late-medieval England: frequently, each point is illustrated by four or more examples drawn from a broad variety of sources, from literary texts to archival documents, and in all three of the languages of medieval England: Middle English, Anglo-Norman and Latin. Three cultural contexts are favored in which to understand the senses: the moral/spiritual connections the senses were understood to have, their place in natural philosophical or scientific thought, and the physiological/medical conceptualization of the senses (p. 16). In this way, in Chapter 2 he describes how nuns' movements were controlled by the Council of London in 1268 in order to preserve their innocence as the senses were portals of the sins, but he also points to a Lollard sermon from the late fourteenth century that demonstrated how the senses can be used for good (p. 17); he describes Walter Burley's examination of the process of vision (pp. 21–2); and he discusses the Salernitan question of why someone who eats cumin remains pale even though the spice is hot and humid (pp. 22–3).

Each chapter in the first section describes a wide range of conceptions that medieval English culture brought to bear on one of the senses. The chapter on touch, for example, deals with connotations in quotidian practice of the right or left hand, medieval names for the fingers, the importance of gestures, the significance of touching (required when making an arrest) or not touching (women, lepers, Jews), corporal punishment, the morality of soft things, kissing, the transference of holiness touch, and the habit of touching objects for their supposed powers. All of this is part of a conceptual framework within which social functions are defined and sensory communities achieved. Some of these groups—elite households—are the subject of the second part of the book because very full documentation exists for them in a way it does not for estates below the aristocracy. They are described here in fascinating and rich detail. In Chapter 11, for example, the Harleian household regulations of the late fifteenth century and the Second Northumberland Household Book are examined for the instruction they provided to the gentleman usher, a servant with a particularly honorary position, for the daily routine and ceremonies of some great households. These documents are later supplemented by the wardrobe accounts of the third Duke of Buckingham (d. 1521) and the *Inventory of Henry VIII*. The regulations for the gentleman usher demonstrate the way an environment of reverence was created for the lord in which textiles and cushions produced a softness that traveled with the peripatetic court as part of the sensory impact of lordship. Objects to be touched by the lord were fetishized by the servants in gestures forbidden to them in connection with the lord's person: they were instructed to kiss the cushions the lord would kneel on during mass (pp. 250–1), or the cloth with which the lord was to serve during the Maundy ceremony (p. 253). Changes can also be seen in sensory display: by the mid-sixteenth century paintings and maps fixed on the walls were part of the visual fashion rather than textiles to be carried with the traveling court. In Henry VIII's household, the smell of cinnamon was used in the chapel for its associations with sanctity, but other odors were demonstrations of power. Sets of perfume became part of the king's essential projection of monarchy.

The conceptualization and shaping of sensory experience in the Middle Ages in theory and practice are subjects that will occupy medievalists and historians of the senses with increasing specialization and refinement in the coming years. What the two works surveyed here (and others like them, such as the 2002 volume of *Micrologus*) demonstrate is how essential the study of the sensorium is to a more complete understanding of the Middle Ages. But at the same time, how essential the Middle Ages are to the writing of a sensory history that raises the claim of being comprehensive.

EXHIBITION REVIEWS

Senses & Society   VOLUME 4, ISSUE 3   REPRINTS AVAILABLE   PHOTOCOPYING   © BERG 2009
    PP 375–378   DIRECTLY FROM THE   PERMITTED BY   PRINTED IN THE UK
    PUBLISHERS   LICENSE ONLY

Honest Threads

By Iris Häussler. Curated by Mona Filip as an offsite project of The Koffler Centre for the Arts. Honest Ed's Department Store, Toronto, January 22–March 8, 2009.

Sarah Aranha

This blouse originally belonged to my mother, Anna Aversa, and I inherited it after her death in 2005; since her passing I have found my memories of her fading away and so I am trying my hardest to hold onto any piece of her that I can. This blouse reminds me of her, and is a bit mysterious at the same time; I don't ever remember her wearing it and I wasn't able to find any photos of her in it either. While this blouse has a history of its own, one that I may never uncover; I myself am creating a new history for it, as it completes my wardrobe.

Teresa Aversa (detail from *Honest Threads*)

Sarah Aranha is an artist, critic, and Exhibitions Coordinator for Wedge Curatorial Projects, Toronto. sarah.aranha@gmail.com

The above passage is one of about 200 narratives similarly recounting the significance of a beloved item of clothing. Torontonians who responded to a call for submissions tell the stories behind a pair of black trousers, a prom dress, a military uniform, a chef's jacket, and a Moroccan dress, among a diversity of other

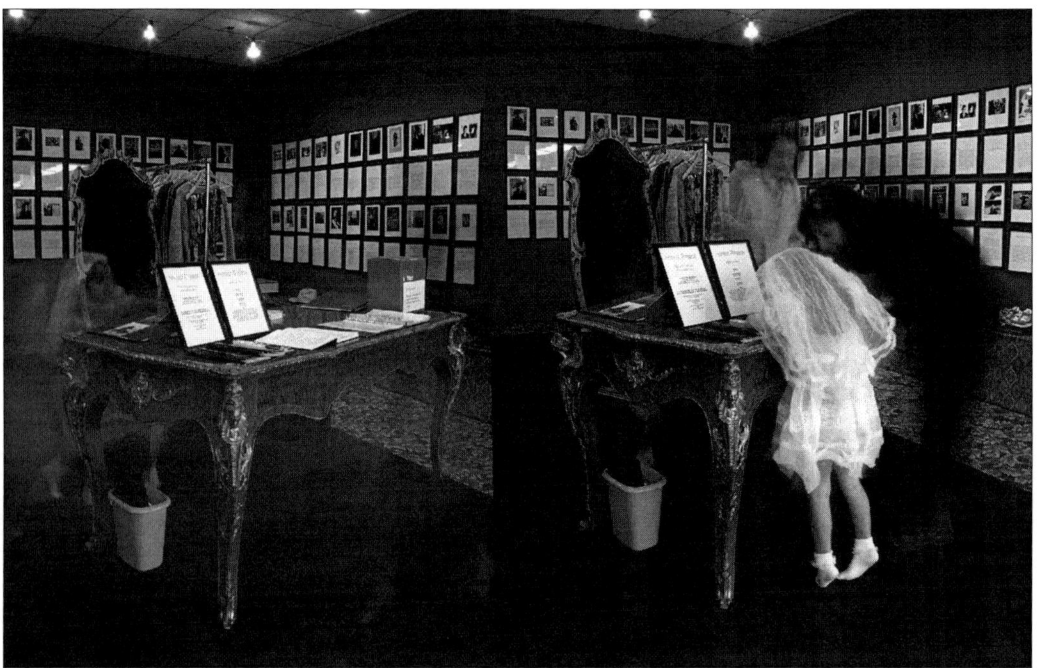

Figure 1
Iris Häussler, *Honest Threads*, 2009, installation views. Photograph by Isaac Applebaum, courtesy of the artist and The Koffler Centre for the Arts.

garments. Candidly written, some are short and to the point, while others paint a picture of faraway countries and long-lost friends. All the stories feature a photo of the owner wearing the item and line the walls of Iris Häussler's installation, *Honest Threads* (2009).

Set up as a vintage secondhand store of sorts, *Honest Threads* is housed within Honest Ed's Department Store, a 160,000 square foot bargain store in operation since 1948. A Toronto landmark, it is a beacon for newcomers to the city as its low prices and door-crasher deals provide families and students alike with affordable basics such as clothing, kitchenware, and groceries. Its gaudy exterior – made up of hundreds of bulbs that spell out "Honest Ed's" in bright lights and corny slogans ("The only thing crooked about Honest Ed's is the floor!") – holds a special place in the heart of Torontonians. One would be hard-pressed to find someone who has never had some kind of interaction with the bargain store.

Honest Threads uses the site as a point of departure. Charting personal and collective histories is a central theme in Häussler's artistic practice, and the exhibition explores these ideas by using clothes as a conduit for memory and storytelling. When people submitted their stories to Häussler they also donated that particular item of clothing for the duration of the exhibition. On display in the center of the small space in the men's department where *Honest Threads* is installed all of the various ballerina costumes, bolero jackets, T-shirts, and high-school sweaters hang on easily accessible clothing racks. Unlike the jeans and shorts strewn in bins throughout the regular aisles of Honest Ed's, visitors are welcome to borrow the clothes in the installation for up to five days. As the press release states, the project promotes "experiencing both literally and psychologically what it is like to 'walk in someone else's shoes'."

The exhibition resists being a static document of the past. Rather, there is a dynamic energy in the space, as the narratives and memories are made real through the presence of the clothing items. Removed from the context in which the jackets, tap shoes, and cocktail dresses were once worn and thus remembered, they are neatly arranged on hangers and are physically there to be felt, smelled, and even tried on if one may so desire. Häussler sees this as a "haptic experience," in which something intangible or distant is made immediate and alive. By presenting the clothes alongside the stories, each piece of clothing oscillates between being a precious artifact of a personal history and a utilitarian object that still has potential for further use.

This oscillation, ultimately, is the strength of *Honest Threads*. Jennifer Fisher, in her writing on relational aesthetics and the haptic sense, demarcates the difference between the visual and haptic sensorial modes. She states that "where the visual sense permits a transcendent, distant and arguably disconnected point-of-view, the haptic sense functions by contiguity, contact and resonance."[1] Häussler's careful mediation of these two aspects of the installation forces visitors to deal with what they see and what they feel simultaneously. The text-laden walls at first seem to estrange visitors from each other and the objects in the room. The many anecdotes and remembrances are absorbing and, combined with the introspective mood set by the warm lighting and plush red interior, it is easy to compulsively read each story on the walls. The distance between the owner's memory and the reality of the exhibition is bridged by the physical availability of the clothing about which one has read. Being able to touch the patent leather shoes that belonged to Ed Mirvish, founder of Honest Ed's, to feel the small hole in the trouser seam where someone once hid a key, to see how a fancy hat fits on one's head, all serves to anchor the experience in the present. As people begin to talk to each other and identify specific pieces of clothing from a story that struck them in particular, Fisher's notion of resonance and contact as attributes of the haptic become clear. Connections are made between friends and strangers, between the past and the present, and, as participants try the apparel on, storylines are extended into unknown territory.

It is all these layers that contribute to the depth of *Honest Threads*. Honest Ed's continues to serve as a literal and psychological meeting point for people of the city, and the clothes in the red room on the second floor allows their stories to be exchanged. The embroidered jackets, knitted ponchos, hockey jerseys, and christening gowns are special items from our collective wardrobe, markers of times and places past, while remaining open to the endless possibilities of the day.

Figure 2
Iris Häussler, *Honest Threads*, 2009, detail of photographs and texts. Photograph courtesy of the artist and The Koffler Centre for the Arts.

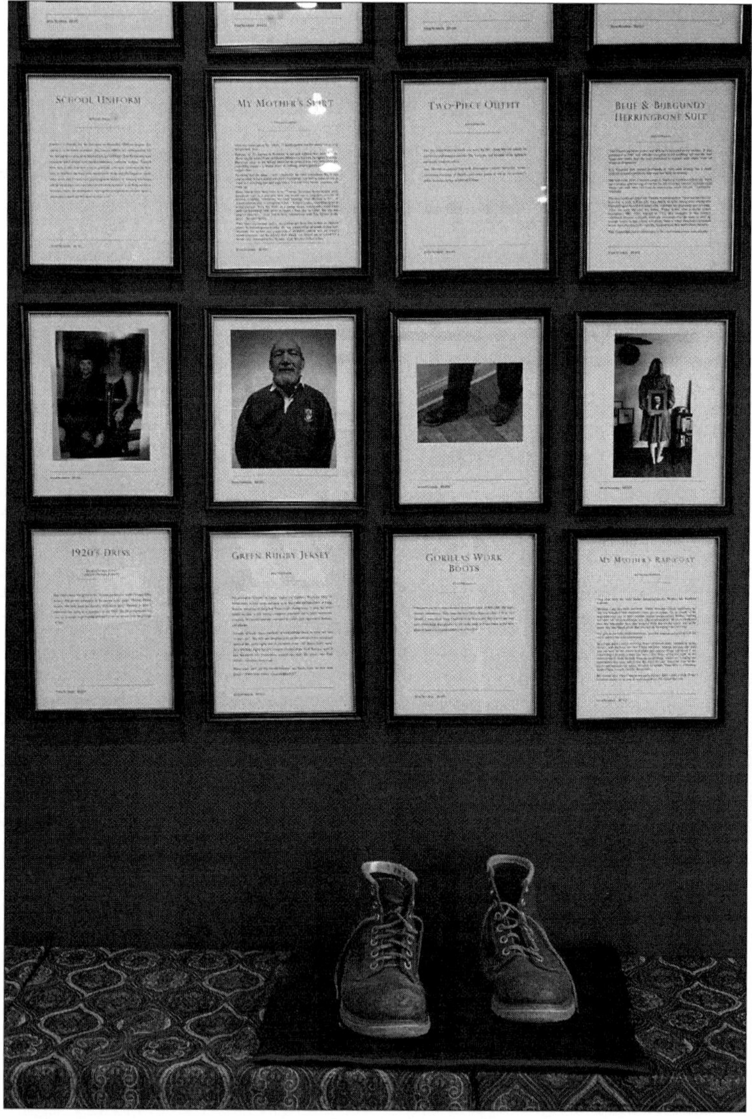

Note

1. Jennifer Fisher, "Relational Sense: Towards a Haptic Aesthetics," *Parachute* #87, July/August/September, 1997, p. 6.

Senses & Society VOLUME 4, ISSUE 3 REPRINTS AVAILABLE PHOTOCOPYING © BERG 2009
PP 379–386 DIRECTLY FROM THE PERMITTED BY PRINTED IN THE UK
PUBLISHERS LICENSE ONLY

Touching Art
Touching You

Royal Cornwall Museum, Truro, UK.
July 26–October 4, 2008.

Harriet Hawkins

Harriet Hawkins is
an AHRC Research
Fellow in the School of
Geography, University
of Exeter. She is
currently preparing
publications from
her doctoral thesis
on the geographies
of contemporary art
practice, including the
sensory experience of
installation art.
h.hawkins@exeter.ac.uk

The sensory experiences of hearing, smelling, and, most importantly, touch are at the heart of BlindArt's mandate, a charity inaugurated in 2004 to support art created by sighted and visually-impaired artists and to promote aesthetic experience beyond the visual. Following the success of their international touring exhibitions, "Sense & Sensuality" (2005 and 2006), a portion of BlindArt's permanent collection was exhibited at the Royal Cornwall Museum under the title "Touching Art Touching You."[1]

In this modest exhibition, paintings lined the walls and a series of sculptural works posed on free-standing plinths. The steady hum emitted by Tine Bech and Sam Woolf's sound/touch work *Echidna* (2002) – a nest of black copper wires – provided the show's overall ambience. Tapping the wires with one's fingertips resulted in a staccato high-pitched tone, while placing one's palm on the sculpture elicited a prolonged light-saber-like sound, breaking the monotony of the hum. Moving through the exhibition involved negotiating these waves of sounds. Joining the hum were the crooning

Senses & Society DOI 10.2752/174589209X12464528172175

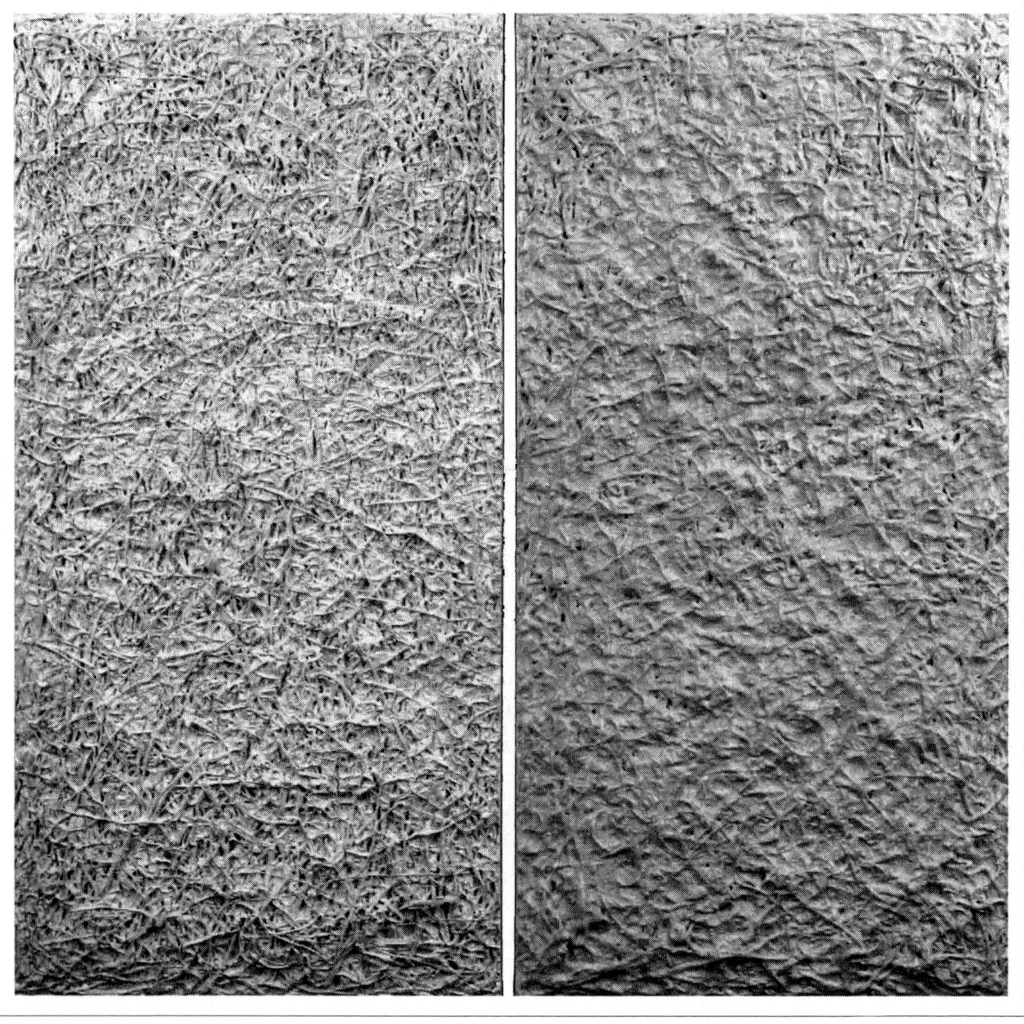

Figure 1
Michael Cahillane, *Chalk and Cheese* (c.2005), mixed media. Photograph courtesy of BlindArt Permanent Collection © BlindArt.

tones of an Elvis song, the soundtrack to *Elvis (What Do You Want Me to Do?)* (c.2005), a video by Nigel Foster, and the tinny mechanical tinkle of music boxes in Alexandra Conil-Lacoste's *Musical Hirst* (c.2005). Circulating around the gallery, caught on currents of air, were wafts of seven essential oils from *Symphonie des Parfums* (2007), also by Conil-Lacoste; the scents waxed and waned as visitors opened and shut the multi-colored boxes.

Despite these sensory offerings, the exhibition did not forget the eye. Instead, there was an, at times, less-than-nuanced questioning of vision as authoritarian, complete, and detached. The apparent ease with which some see was problematized in Fiona Zobole's *S1&ht3d* (c.2005), in which she created a long canvas of increasingly unreadable text. A similar line of critique was pursued in Joanna Brendon's *Just Looking* (c.2005), in which the artist assembled

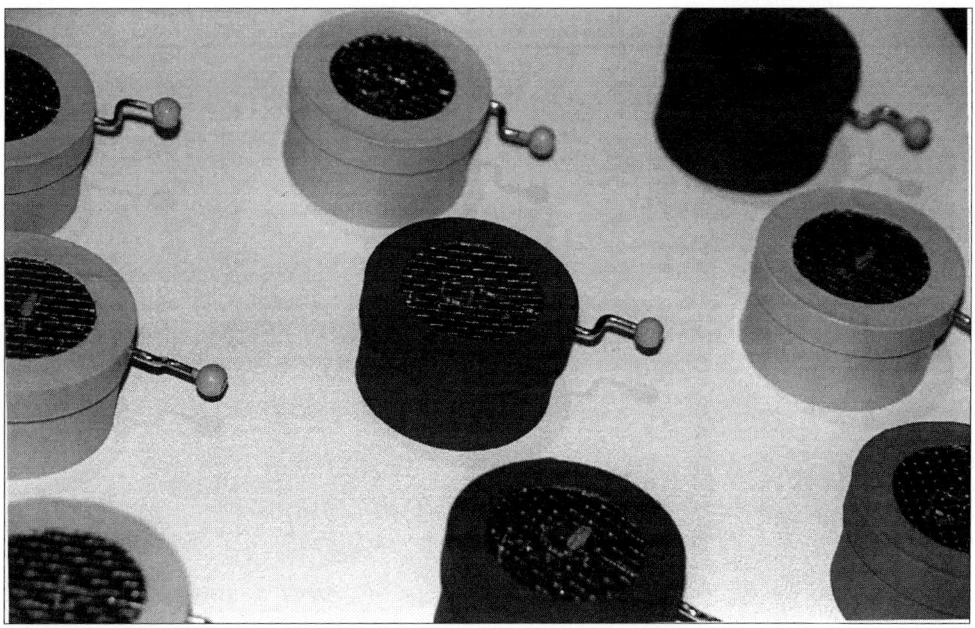

Figure 2
Alexandra Conil-Lacoste, *Musical Hirst* (c.2005), music boxes and wood. Photograph courtesy of BlindArt Permanent Collection © BlindArt.

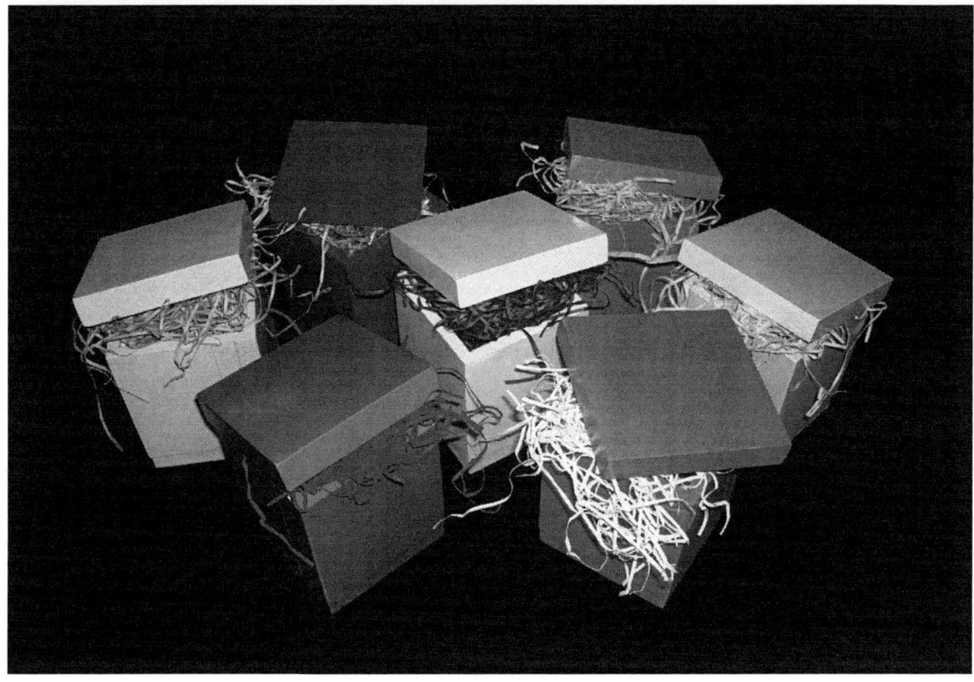

Figure 3
Alexandra Conil-Lacoste, *Symphonie des Parfums* (2007), essential oils, shredded paper, painted wooden boxes. Photograph courtesy of BlindArt Permanent Collection © BlindArt.

an iris of navy blue flocked words on black paper. The thirty-six descriptions of vision – "leer," " glimpse," "gaze," "peep" – were legible only with effort. Across the floor, Natasha Lewer's *Blood Cells* (2005) rendered microscopic platelets and white blood cells large, singular, and solid in ceramic and rich-colored flocking. Beyond these critiques of vision, the exhibition proposed a more general challenge to the museum space as one devoted to sight or, indeed, any particular sense alone.

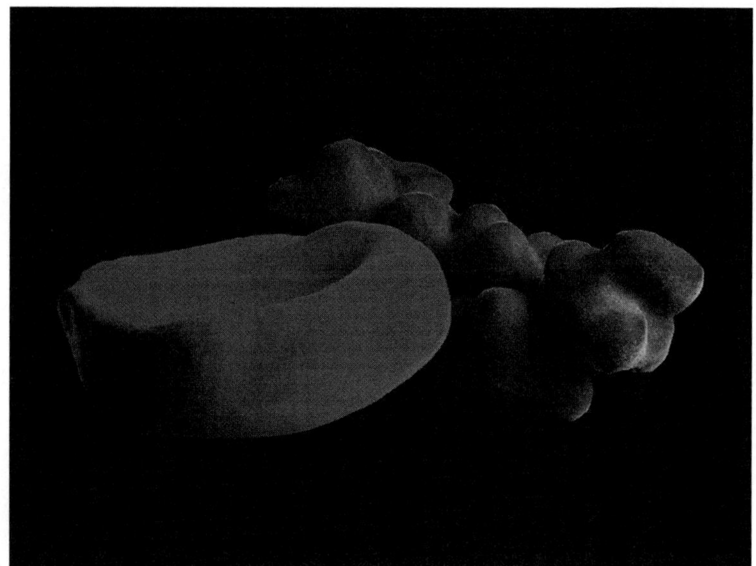

Figure 4
Natasha Lewer, *Blood Cells* (2005), ceramic and flocking. Photograph courtesy of BlindArt Permanent Collection © BlindArt.

Even though the logic of the exhibition was primarily an optical one, it took the form of a haptic visuality. Interestingly, I touched because I could, and because I felt it was expected of me, rather than as an instinctive response compelled by the works' tactility. For example, I did not feel the same sense of wanting to reach out inspired by Meret Oppenheim's lascivious furry cup and saucer, or the curves and hollows of a Barbara Hepworth or Henry Moore sculpture. Instead, I was overly aware of the need to interact, a sense that I was supposed to touch, which at times uncomfortably drifted towards an experience akin to the hands-on science museum. But in these enforced interactions I become acutely aware of the particular modalities of touch. Most effective in drawing these out were the paired canvases *Chalk and Cheese* (2005) by Michael Cahillane where different painted "whites" translated into different textures. *Cheese*, a yellowy cream painting with clotted, knotted masses of paint and string, featured a surface that was smoothed over to the touch. The work drew me closer as I shifted from fingertip to palm spread, and eventually, apprehensively, to both hands at once.

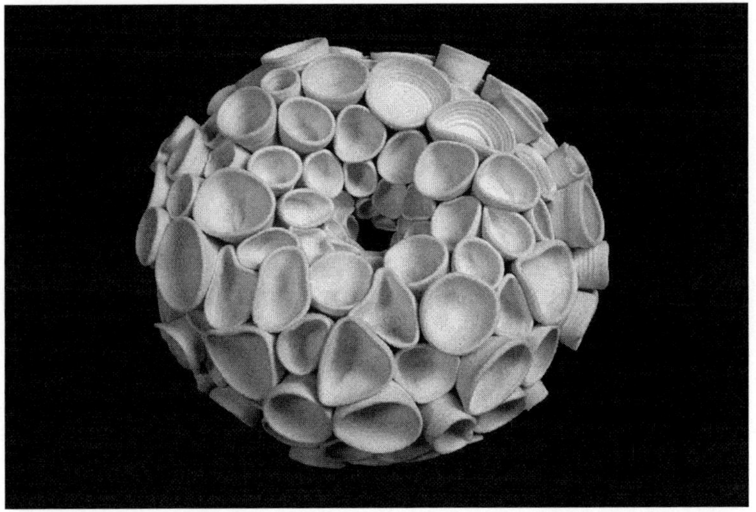

Figure 5
Natasha Lewer, *Barnacles*,
(2005), ceramic and
flocking. Photograph
courtesy of BlindArt
Permanent Collection
© BlindArt.

Approaching still closer I could see the greyish tinge left by the
palms of others. The second panel, *Chalk*, was a clearer, sharper
white. Here my fingertips traced the ridges made by the string and
one could follow a precise line, the passage of which was continually
halted by numerous knobs and bumps.

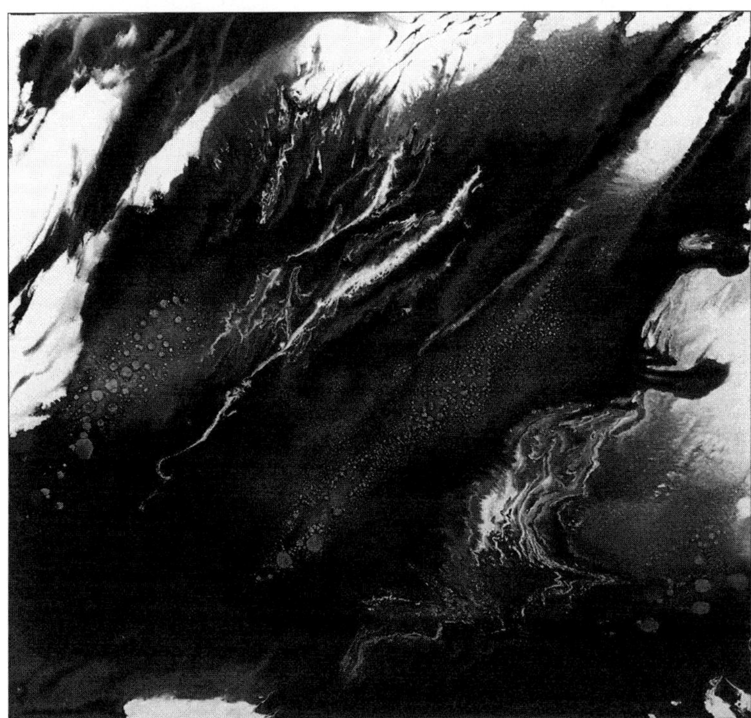

Figure 6
Lyn Lemont Webb, *Ice*
(2005), oil and alkyd resin
on canvas. Photograph
courtesy of BlindArt
Permanent Collection
© BlindArt.

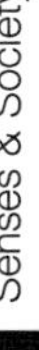

In this transgression of the gallery's visual regime I felt bereft of the disciplinary technologies that normally order my corporeality as a seeing subject. Here, forced to touch, I failed as a haptic subject. I was ill-equipped to know these works, for they called into question the facile assumptions of the all-seeing eye. Should I have shut my eyes, felt with both hands or only one, sensed for textures with fingertip or palm, or even arm or cheek? With eyes closed I felt vulnerable, with eyes open I constantly tried to triangulate divergent sensory impressions. In some cases I was intrigued by how a plush, flocked surface betrayed the cold, hard porcelain form it covered (*Blood Cells*), or was surprised by the softness of what

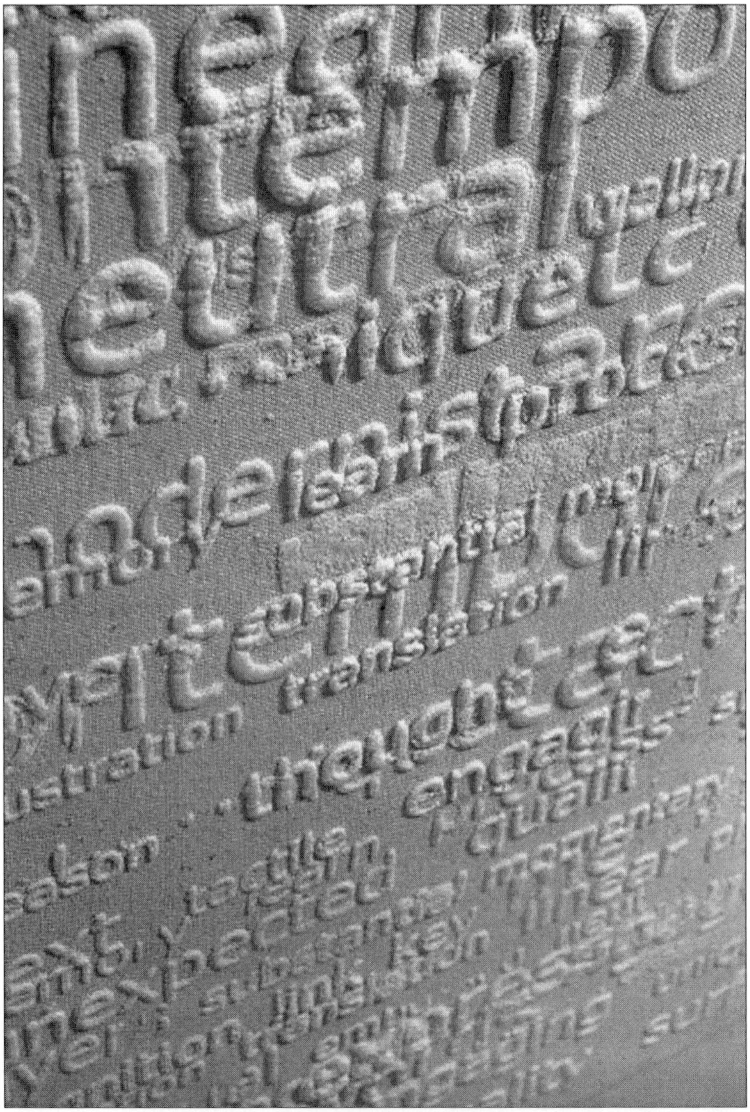

Figure 7
Fiona Zobole, *S1&ht3d* (c.2005), screen-printed text on canvas. Photograph courtesy of BlindArt Permanent Collection © BlindArt.

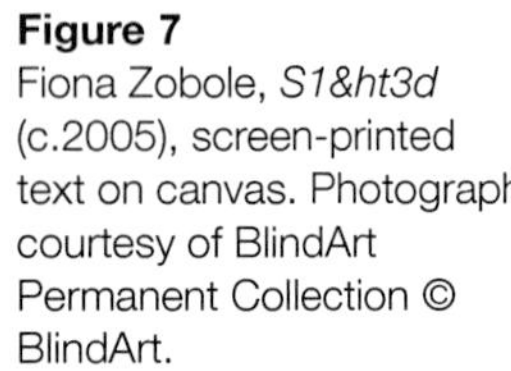

initially seemed brittle and fragile (*Barnacles*, 2005, also by Lewer). Frustration developed when the energy and exuberance visible within paint stokes did not translate beneath my fingers (*Mirror*, c.2005, by Frances Aviva Blane). The fluidity and lucidity evident in the mixing of striking colors in *Ice* (2005), by Lyn Lemont Webb, were lost beneath my palms, where touch found only bubbles and the occasional smooth rubberized surface of pooled resin. It became clear that I did not have the skills needed to comprehend art, or the world, through touch.

Experiencing these works, I came to understand them on a scale keyed to the intimacy of the body – it became important whether a work was as wide as the spread of my arms or as tall as my form. Touching them I entered into a newly intimate, even sensual, space that, at times, reached towards the inter-subjectivity implied by the exhibition's title. "Touching Art Touching You" certainly questioned the modalities of vision, took viewers back to the full sensory definition of "aesthetics," and made visitors aware of a gallery experience constructed on terms other than ocularcentrism. While the subject addressed by the exhibition is still a seeing one, she also hears, smells, and touches, even if it is not entirely clear that she knows how.

Note

1. For further information on BlindArt and their permanent collection please go to their website: www.blindart.net

The Senses & Society

Notes to Contributors

- Articles should be between 4,500 and 8,000 words (but not exceeding 8,000 words in length unless by prior agreement please).
- They must include a 30 word biography of the author(s) and a 200-word abstract and 3 to 5 keywords.
- Interviews should also include an author biography.
- Exhibition and book reviews should be approximately 750 words, with occasional reviews running to 2,500 words.
- The Publishers will require a disk as well as a hard copy of any contributions.

From time to time, *Senses & Society* plans to produce special issues devoted to a single topic with a guest editor. Persons wishing to organize a topical issue are invited to submit a proposal which contains a 500-word description of the topic together with a list of potential contributors and paper subjects. Proposals are accepted only after a review by the Journal editors and in-house editorial staff at Berg Publishers.

Manuscripts

- Manuscripts should be sent electronically in Microsoft Word with accompanying hard copy to:
  David Howes, Managing Editor, The Senses and Society, Department of Sociology and Anthropology, Concordia University, 1455 de Maisonneuve Boulevard West, Montreal, Quebec, Canada H3G 1M8, email: senses@alcor. concordia.ca
- Manuscripts will be acknowledged and entered into the review process discussed below.
- Manuscripts without illustrations will not be returned unless the author provides a self-addressed stamped envelope.
- Submission of a manuscript to the journal will be taken to imply that it is not being considered elsewhere, in the same form, in any language, without the consent of the editor and publisher. It is a condition of acceptance by the editor of a manuscript for publication that the publishers automatically acquire the copyright of the published article throughout the world. Senses & Society does not pay authors for their manuscripts nor does it provide retyping, drawing, or mounting of illustrations.

Style

- US spelling and mechanicals are to be used. Authors are advised to consult The Chicago Manual of Style (15th Edition) as a guideline for style. Webster's Dictionary is our arbiter of spelling. We encourage the use of major subheadings and, where appropriate, second-level subheadings.
- Manuscripts submitted for consideration as an article must contain:
  – a title page with the full title of the article, the author(s) name and address
  – a 30-word biography for each author.
- Do not place the author's name on any other page of the manuscript.

Manuscript Preparation

- Manuscripts must be typed double-spaced (including quotations, notes and references cited), on one side only, with at least one-inch margins on standard paper using a typeface no smaller than 12pts.
- The original manuscript and a copy of the text on disk (please ensure it is clearly marked with the word-processing program that has been used) must be submitted, along with original photographs (to be returned).
- Authors should retain a copy for their records.
- Any necessary artwork must be submitted with the manuscript.

Footnotes

- Footnotes appear as 'Notes' at the end of articles.
- Authors are advised to include footnote material in the text whenever possible.
- Notes are to be numbered consecutively throughout the paper and are to be typed double-spaced at the end of the text
- **(Please do not use any footnoting or end-noting programs which your software may offer as this text becomes irretrievably lost at the typesetting stage.)**

References

- The list of references should be limited to, and inclusive of, those publications actually cited in the text.
- References are to be cited in the body of the text in parentheses with author's last name, the year of original publication, and page number—e.g. (Rouch 1958: 45).
- Titles and publication information appear as 'References' at the end of the article and should be listed alphabetically by author and chronologically for each author.
- References should be written in the following formats:

  Lewis, I.M. and C. Besteman. 1998. "Violence in Somalia: an Exchange." *Cultural Anthropology* 13(1): 100–14.

  Mayer, E. 1992. "Peru in Deep Trouble: Mario Vargas Llosa's 'Inquest in the Andes' Reexamined." In G.E. Marcus (ed.) *Rereading Cultural Anthropology*, pp.181–219. Durham: Duke University Press.

  Stoll, D. 1999. *Rigoberta Menchu and the Story of All Poor Guatemalans*. Boulder: Westview Press.
- Names of journals and publications should appear in full. Film and video information appear as 'Filmography'.
- References cited should be typed double-spaced on a separate page.
- References not presented in the style required will be returned to the author for revision.

Tables

- All tabular material should be part of a separately numbered series of 'Tables'.
- Each table must be typed on a separate sheet and identified by a short descriptive title.
- Footnotes for tables appear at the bottom of the table.
- Marginal notations on manuscripts should indicate approximately where tables are to appear.

Figures

All illustrative material: drawings, maps, diagrams, and photographs should be designated 'Figures'. They must be submitted in a form suitable for publication without redrawing.

- Drawings should be carefully done with India ink on either hard, white, smooth-surfaced board or good quality tracing paper. Ordinarily, computer-generated drawings are not of publishable quality.
- Photographs should be glossy prints and should be numbered on the back to key with captions. Whenever possible, photographs should be 8 × 10 inches.
- The publishers also encourage artwork to be submitted as scanned files (300dpi or above ONLY) on disc or via email.
- All figures should be numbered consecutively.
- All captions should be typed double-spaced on a separate page.
- Marginal notations on manuscripts should indicate approximately where figures are to appear.
- While the editors and publishers will use all reasonable care in protecting all figures submitted, they cannot assume responsibility for their loss or damage. Authors are discouraged from submitting rare or non-replaceable materials. It is the author's responsibility to secure written copyright clearance (for both print and online usage) on all photographs and drawings that are not in the public domain.

Criteria for Evaluation

Senses & Society is a refereed journal. Manuscripts will be accepted only after review by both the editors and anonymous reviewers deemed competent to make professional judgments concerning the quality of the manuscript.

Offprints

On publication, authors will be sent a PDF eprint (with nonprinting watermark) of the final, published version of their article for personal use, and will be able to order a free copy of the issue in which their article appears.

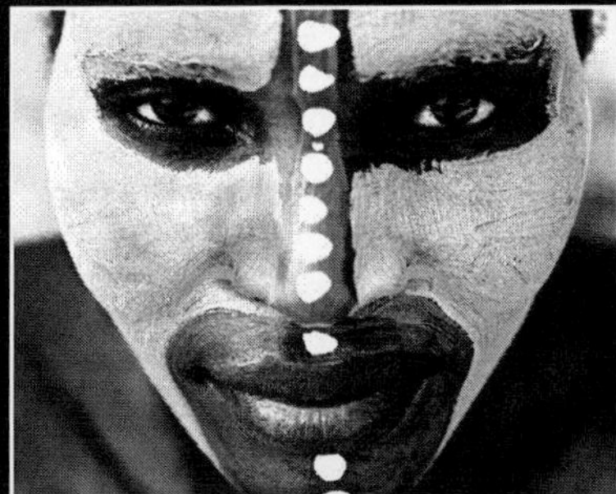
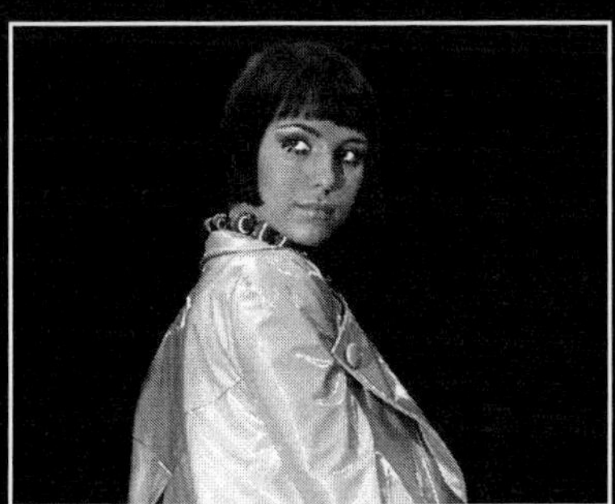
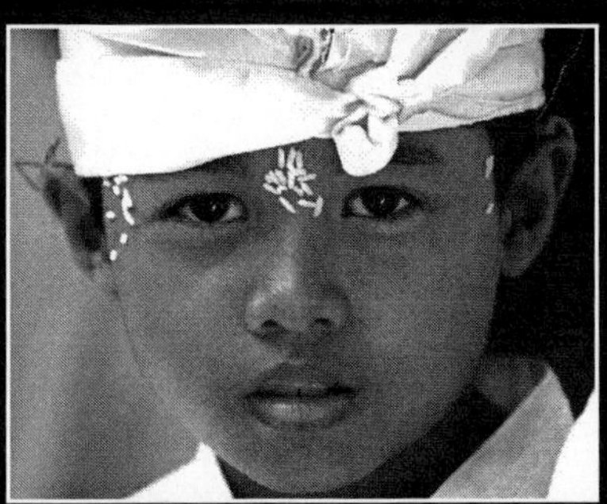
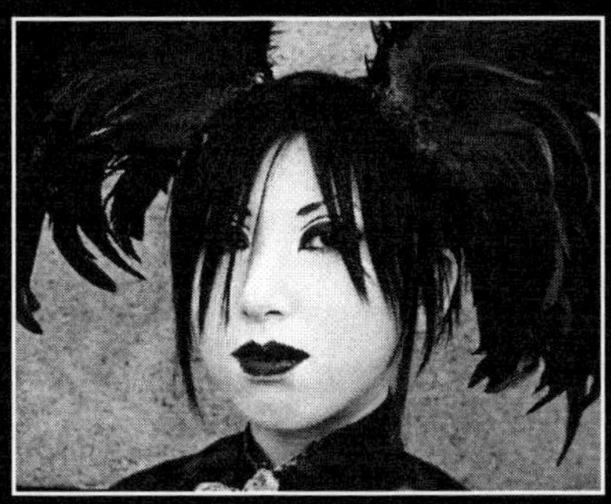